Cardiovascular MRI in Congenital Heart Disease

An Imaging Atlas

Shankar Sridharan · Gemma Price
Oliver Tann · Marina Hughes · Vivek Muthurangu
Andrew M. Taylor

Cardiovascular MRI in Congenital Heart Disease

An Imaging Atlas

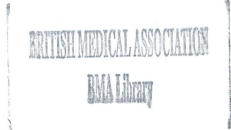

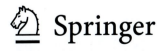 Springer

From:

The Centre for Cardiovascular MR
UCL Institute of Child Health & Great Ormond Street Hospital for Children
Cardiovascular Unit
Great Ormond Street
London WC1N 3JH
UK

Dr. Shankar Sridharan
Locum Consultant Paediatric Cardiologist

Gemma Price
Medical Illustrator

Dr. Oliver Tann
Consultant In Cardiovascular Imaging

Dr. Marina Hughes
Consultant Paediatric Cardiologist
Clinical Lead for CMR

Dr. Vivek Muthurangu
BHF Intermediate Research Fellow

Professor Andrew M. Taylor
Professor of Cardiovascular Imaging
Director – Centre for Cardiovascular MR

ISBN 978-3-540-69836-4   eISBN 978-3-540-69837-1
DOI 10.1007/978-3-540-69837-1

Springer Heidelberg Dordrecht London New York

Library of Congress Control Number: 2009938029

© Springer-Verlag Berlin Heidelberg 2010

Cover design: eStudio Calamar Figueres Berlin

Printed on acid-free paper

9 8 7 6 5 4 3 2 1 0

springer.com

Preface

The last 10 years has seen explosive expansion of the number of centres performing cardiovascular magnetic resonance (CMR) imaging. The majority of this expansion has been in the field of adult ischaemic imaging, but congenital heart disease remains one of the main indications for CMR. Importantly, the greatly improved survival of patients with congenital heart disease gives us a burgeoning adult population living with the sequelae of the disease (grown-up congenital heart disease – GUCH).

Without previous experience or formal training, the interpretation of CMR images of patients with congenital heart disease can be difficult. The main aim of this book is to create a portable resource that offers efficient access to high-quality MR (and where appropriate, CT) images of the common congenital and structural heart abnormalities. We hope that by providing key images for each condition and a clear interpretation of the MR appearances, we will improve the reader's understanding of the conditions, facilitate their interpretation of images and optimise the planning of the imaging protocols during their own practice of congenital CMR.

As with any publication from a single institution, the contents of this book represent our own practice. We have not written a definitive or exhaustive description of the conditions. However, we hope that we have produced a factual, simple and eye-pleasing guide for fellows training in CMR, radiographers and technicians performing CMR scans, physician users of CMR, and perhaps those few in adult ischaemic practice, who may need the occasional aide memoir for incidental findings!

We hope that you will find this book useful in your everyday practice and learning.

Shankar Sridharan
Gemma Price
Oliver Tann
Marina Hughes
Vivek Muthurangu
Andrew Taylor

London, UK

Contents

1 Technical Considerations

Paediatric Challenges

- The usual technical difficulties faced when performing a cardiac MR examination are further amplified when imaging small children
- Optimal image quality may be compromised because of
  - The smaller size of structures
  - Faster heart rates
  - The reduced time for image acquisition (inability or difficulty with breath-holding)
- The imaging protocol should be prioritised to obtain the most crucial diagnostic information, in case the patient's cooperation is limited

1. Spatial Resolution

Smaller field-of-views (FOVs) and the use of thinner slices are required to image small anatomical structures.

This leads to increased image resolution, but a corresponding reduction in signal:noise (S/N) ratio. This can be compensated by

- Increasing the number of acquisitions – (disadvantage: increase in scan time)
- Removing parallel imaging features – (disadvantage: increase in scan time)
- Using a coarser matrix, to increase diagnostic image quality, albeit at the cost of reduced resolution

2. Appropriate Coil Selection

Appropriate coil selection is important to maximise S/N ratio.

- A dedicated extremity (knee coil) should be used in neonates or very small children.
- A transmit/receive coil can reduce noise and increase S/N ratio.
- If the child is too large for this, then a body matrix and spine coil combination achieves good results.

3. Faster Heart Rates

Faster heart rates in small children result in a short R-R period.

- For sequences where repetition times (TR) are longer than the R-R period, gating, using the second or third R wave as the trigger facilitates more time for the appropriate recovery of longitudinal magnetisation.
- For cine-imaging, reducing the number of phase encode steps in each frame will decrease the acquisition period for each frame, improving temporal resolution and image sharpness. However, this increases scan times.

4. Strategies to Reduce Motion Artefact

- Play therapy or pre-examination visits to the scanner can help a child overcome any anxiety and improve in-magnet stillness.
- Installing a DVD/Video system is a worthwhile investment to promote prolonged distraction and cooperation.
- For children who have difficulty breath-holding, images can be acquired during free breathing. Additionally:
  - Use manual shimming techniques, as they are essential to minimise flow artefacts, particularly on balanced SSFP sequences
  - Increase the number of acquisitions (NEX) from 1 to 3
  - Use respiratory compensation methods to acquire data, e.g. use of navigator echoes, phase re-ordering algorithms.
  - Acquire data using real time imaging sequences (where imaging systems allow).

5. Contrast Administration in Children

For angiography, we use 0.2–0.4 mL/kg of Dotarem, (Guerbet, Paris) which corresponds to 0.1–0.2 mmol/kg. All Gadolinium contrast agents need to be given in accordance with Institutional and National guidelines to avoid nephrogenic sytemic fibrosis (NSF). For further information on this, see the UK Royal College of Radiologists document on this subject: http://www.rcr.ac.uk/docs/radiology/pdf/BFCR0714_Gadolinium_NSF_guidanceNov07.pdf

6. Consider Alternative Imaging Strategies

CT is potentially useful if MR assessment is limited or hampered by technical restraints.

2   MR Imaging Under GA

Indications for General Anaesthesia (GA) for Paediatric MR

Practice varies throughout the world. However, most centres in the UK will perform cardiovascular MR under general anaesthetic (GA) for children under the age of 7 years.

General Safety Issues Specific to Paediatric Cardiac Imaging

- Patient metal checked and the safety questionnaire performed with parents before the child is anaesthetised.
- Senior cardiac anaesthetist continuously present in every case.
- Full monitoring: pulse oximetry, end-tidal gas analysis, ECG and non-invasive BP.
- Wrap the patient in gamgee or blankets to keep him or her warm.
- Ten metre circle breathing system needed, to link the patient to anaesthetist in MR control room.
- Breath-holding in passive expiration, controlled by breaking the circuit in the control room.
- The large dead space prohibits low flow anaesthesia.
- Reversal of anaesthesia and extubation in CMR induction room. Ensure that the team is aware of the cardiac arrest procedure.

Importantly, the child MUST be withdrawn from the MR room for resuscitation. Metallic objects such as resuscitation trolley MUST NOT be brought into the scanning room.

Environmental and Physical Constraints

Performing general anaesthesia (GA) in a magnetic resonance (MR) environment is challenging for many reasons

- During the scan, there is limited access to the child and ventilation equipment.
- Care is required for staff and patient safety with regard to ferromagnetic equipment.
- There is a potential for RF interference with monitoring equipment.

Technical Factors Specific to MR in Infants and Small Children

- Prolonged, multiple breath holds are required. This can cause hypoxia. Adequate pause for ventilation control between breath holds is required.
- A reliable ECG is vital for gating during image acquisition.
- Monitor patient temperature closely. The low ambient temperature in MR scanning room produces a hypothermia risk, particularly for small infants.

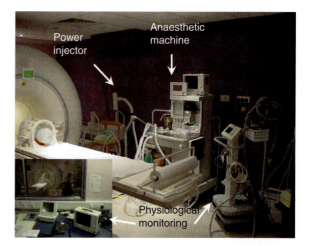

Fig. 2.1. Photography showing one of our dedicated paediatric cardiac MR labs. Inset, control room with monitoring equipment and long anaesthetic tubing to enable the anaesthetist to sit in the controlroom during MR scanning

3 Imaging Protocol

Table 3.1 Suggested imaging protocols for given conditions

Conditions	Scout	Axial BB	Vent cines				CE-MRA				Flow				LGE	Perfusion	Notes
			VLA	4-Ch	AV	SA stack	PA	Ao	SVC	3D SSFP	RVOT Cines	LVOT cines	PA	Ao			
Shunts ASD, SVD, AVSD, VSD	✓	✓	✓	✓	✓	✓	✓	✓	✓	±	✓	✓	✓	✓			Consider AVSD as complex CHD. CE MRA ± for VSD
Valvar AS, AI, MR, MS	✓	✓	✓	✓	✓	✓	✓	✓			±	✓	±	✓	±		
Aorta Coarctation, rings and slings, Marfan	✓	✓	✓	✓	✓	✓	✓	✓		✓	±	✓	±	✓			ECG-gated CT indicated for coarctation stent assessment
RVOT/PA PS, ToF, PA, TGA, truncus	✓	✓	✓	✓	✓	✓	✓	✓		✓	✓	✓	✓	✓	±		ECG-gated CT indicated for stent assessment
Cardiomyopathy HCM, DCM, non compaction	✓	✓	✓	✓	✓	✓	✓	✓			±	✓	±	✓	✓	±	
Coronary arteries Anomalous, ALCAPA, Kawasaki	✓	✓	✓	✓	✓	✓		✓		✓		✓	±	±	✓	±	Use thin slice 3D SSFP ECG-gated coronary CT indicated for identifying stenoses
Complex CHD DORV, DILV, CCTGA, HLHS, BCPC, Fontan, TCPC, Ebstein	✓	✓	✓	✓	✓	✓	✓	✓	±	✓	✓	✓	✓	✓	±	±	Delayed CE MRA essential for BCPC (Glenn), Fontan and TCPC circulations. LGE and stress perfusion may be useful in some

Table 3.2 Imaging protocol (standard sequences and views in the order of workflow)

	Sequence	Planning	1° Purpose	2° Purpose
Scout	Single shot bSSFP images	3 Images in all 3 orthogonal planes	Iso-centering of the heart in the scanner	
Axial stack	Respiratory-navigated, ECG-gated, "black-blood" images (HASTE or TSE). Contiguous axial slices	Coverage from liver to neck. Include aortic arch & proximal branches. Include systemic & pulmonary veins	Planning subsequent cine imaging planes	Provides a map of thoracic anatomy
Ventricular long-axis (RVLA/LVLA)	Breath-held, ECG-gated, bSSFP cine images	From axial stack. Place perpendicular plane through long axis of ventricle, from mid-atrioventricular (AV) valve to ventricular apex	Planning the true 4-chamber image	Assessment of anterior & inferior myocardium, AV valves, ventricular sizes
AV valves	Breath-held, ECG-gated, bSSFP cine image	From axial stack. Place perpendicular plane parallel to, & on apical side of AV. Check that orientation is parallel to the vertical axis of the AV valves on RVLA & LVLA views	Planning the 4-chamber and LV outflow tract (LVOT) images	Subjective evaluation of AV valve function
4-Chamber view	Breath-held, ECG-gated, bSSFP cine image	From AV valves view. Place perpendicular plane across both AV valve orifices. From LVLA cine check that this plane passes through mid-mitral valve and LV apex. From RVLA check that the plane passes through mid-tricuspid valve and RV apex	Subjective assessment of atrial size, biventricular size & function, ventricular wall motion, AV valve regurgitation	Planning short axis (SA) stack
SA stack	Breath-held, ECG-gated, bSSFP cine image	From end-diastolic frame of 4-chamber cine. Place perpendicular plane at hingepoints of both AV valves, with special care to include the entire basal ventricular blood pool. From VLA views, check that the first slice is perpendicular to AV valve hingepoints. Contiguous slices are then placed to cover the entire ventricular mass to the apex	Provides the images required for segmentation of ventricular volumes	Assessment of the ventricular septum, ventricular myocardial morphology & wall motion abnormalities, outflow tracts

Table 3.2 (continued)

	Sequence	Planning	1° Purpose	2° Purpose
MR angiography	Breath-held, not ECG-gated Gadolinium injection 0.2–0.4 mL/kg Infants: injection rate 2 mL/s with 5 mL flush. Older children: injection rate 3 mL/s, 10 mL flush	Isotropic voxels (1.1–1.6 mm). Planned on axial HASTE stack, for coronal-orientated raw data. Include antero-posterior chest wall and lungs. Image acquisition triggered with bolus-tracking to ensure maximum signal in structure of interest. Two acquisitions routinely acquired, with no interval in young children, or a 15 s interval in older children	Angiographic views of large and small thoracic vessels. Images less subject to artifact caused by low velocity or turbulent flow. The second pass acquisition allows assessment of systemic and pulmonary venous anatomy	Subjective determination of preferential blood flow. Can be expanded to perform time-resolved angiography or 4-dimensional angiography
3D bSSFP	Free breathing, respiratory navigated, ecg-gated. Data acquisition optimised to occur in diastole. Signal improved following gadolinium injection & in tachycardic pts by triggering acquisition every second beat. Acquisition time 8–15 min	Planned on axial HASTE stack for sagittal orientation of raw data. Isotropic voxels (1.1–1.6 mm). Respiratory navigator placed mid-right dome of diaphragm, avoiding cardiac region of interest	Provides high-resolution images of intracardiac anatomy, including coronary arteries. Allows multiplanar reformatting	Planning further imaging planes in patients with complex anatomy
LV outflow tract	Breath-held, ECG-gated, bSSFP cine image	From the AV valves cine. Place a perpendicular plane through basal aortic valve and mid-mitral valve orifice. Check that orientation passes through LV apex using LVLA cine. Cross-cut this view to obtain two orthogonal cine views of LVOT	Outflow tract morphology. Subjective assessment of semilunar valve function	Planning phase contrast velocity mapping. Planning "enface" view of semilunar valve
RV outflow tract	Breath-held, ECG-gated, bSSFP cine image	From axial stack. Place perpendicular plane through the pulmonary trunk. Cross-cut this view to obtain two orthogonal cine views of RVOT	Outflow tract morphology. Subjective assessment of semilunar valve function	Planning phase contrast velocity mapping. Planning "enface" view of semilunar valve
Great vessel flow	Non-breath held, ECG-gated Through-plane phase contrast velocity mapping	From the orthogonal outflow tract images. Place a perpendicular plane across the vessel of interest. Place plane just distal to valve leaflets in systole, to avoid turbulent areas of flow. Optimise velocity encoding to maximize accuracy and prevent aliasing	Vessel flow volume. Calculate regurgitant fractions (RF%). Validate ventricular stroke volume measurements	Calculate pulmonary blood flow to systemic blood flow ratio (Qp:Qs). Evaluate presence and location of shunts. Calculate flow velocity

4 Normal Anatomy-Axial

The transverse or axial plane is useful for studying morphology and the relationships of the four cardiac chambers and the pericardium.

Images (**a**) through (**f**) show axial planes in a head to foot direction.

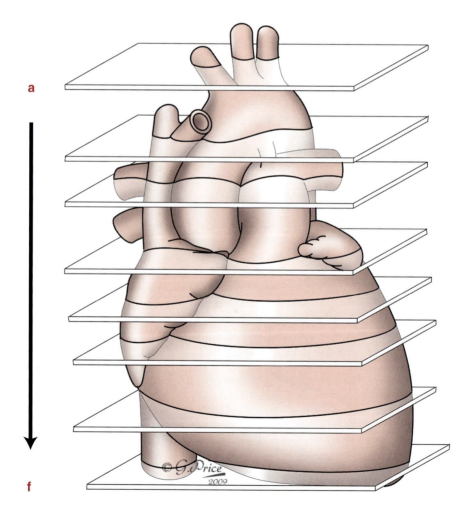

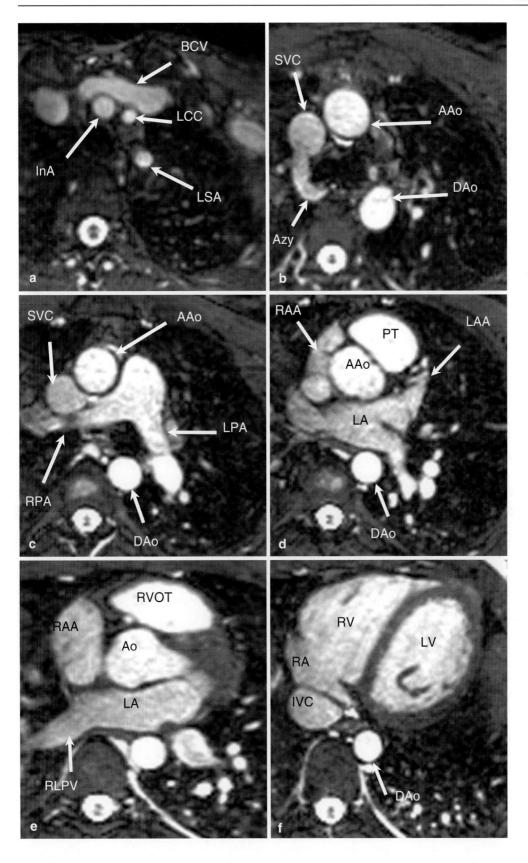

5   Normal Anatomy-Coronal

Frontal or coronal images are most useful for investigation of the LVOT, of the left atrium, and the pulmonary veins.

Images (**a**) through (**f**) show coronal planes through the heart in an apex-to-base direction.

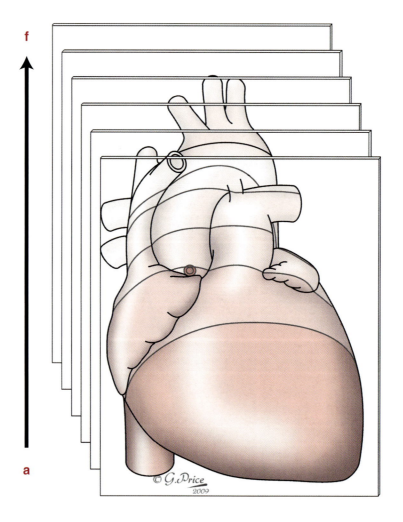

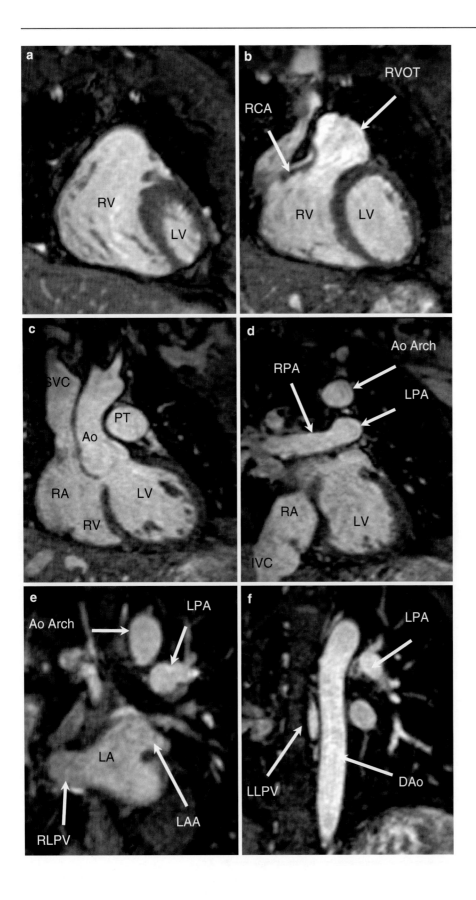

6 Normal Anatomy-Sagittal

Saggital images can be used to study the connections between the ventricles and the great vessels.

Images (**a**) through (**f**) show saggital planes through the heart in a right-to-left direction.

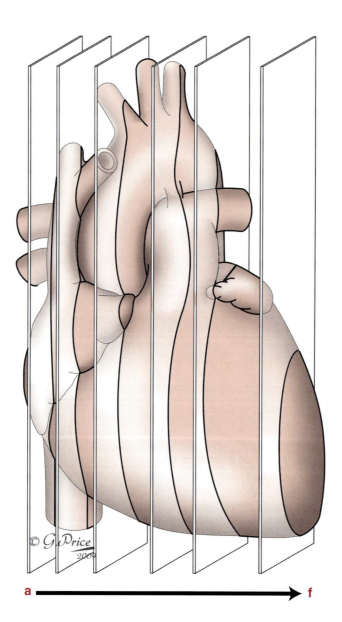

a ➝ f

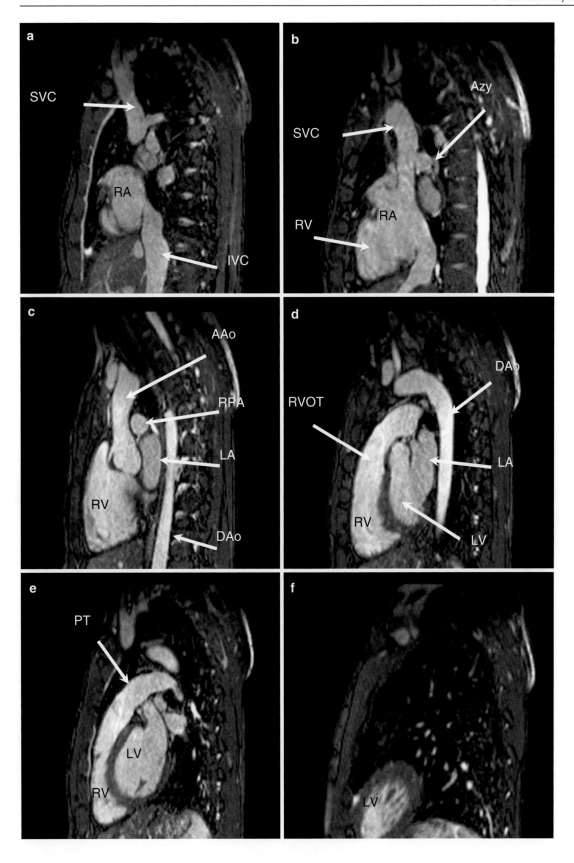

7   Image Planes-Ventricles

Planned using HASTE axial stack, and acquired using a b-SSFP sequence.

These figures illustrate the process with normal anatomy. The same principles are used for patients with any ventricular arrangement.

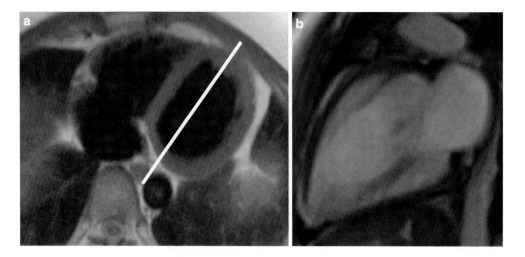

Fig. 7.1. The LV vertical long axis plane (LVLA) is aligned using the axial plane, through the mitral valve and the LV apex, which may be on a separate more inferior slice

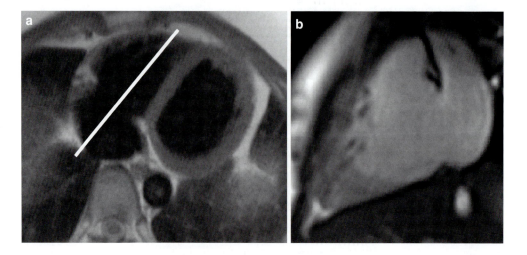

Fig. 7.2. The RV vertical long axis plane (RVLA) is aligned using the axial plane, through the tricuspid valve and the RV anterior wall – apex

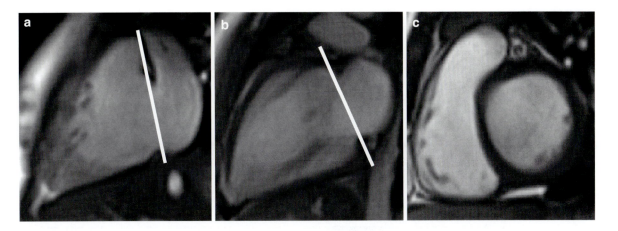

Fig. 7.3. The short axis plane (SA) is aligned using the VLA views and the axial plane, and is perpendicular to both

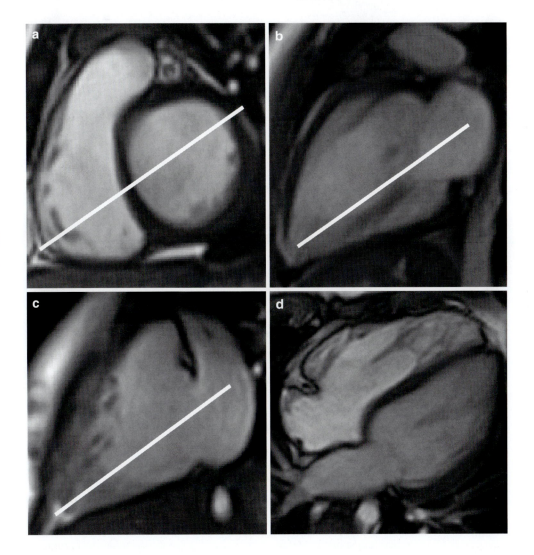

Fig. 7.4. The 4-chamber view is planned using the SA and the VLA views. A perpendicular line is placed through the anterior mitral valve papillary muscle and the apex of the RV in the SA, and then adjusted to intersect the LV and RV apices in VLA views

8   Imaging Planes-Left Ventricular Outflow Tract

Planned and acquired using b-SSFP sequence.

LVOT view useful for septal hypertrophy and LVOT obstruction in HCM.

Aortic valve plane used for through-plane Ao flow, and valve morphology.

These figures illustrate the process with normal anatomy. The same principles are used for patients with any ventricular arrangement.

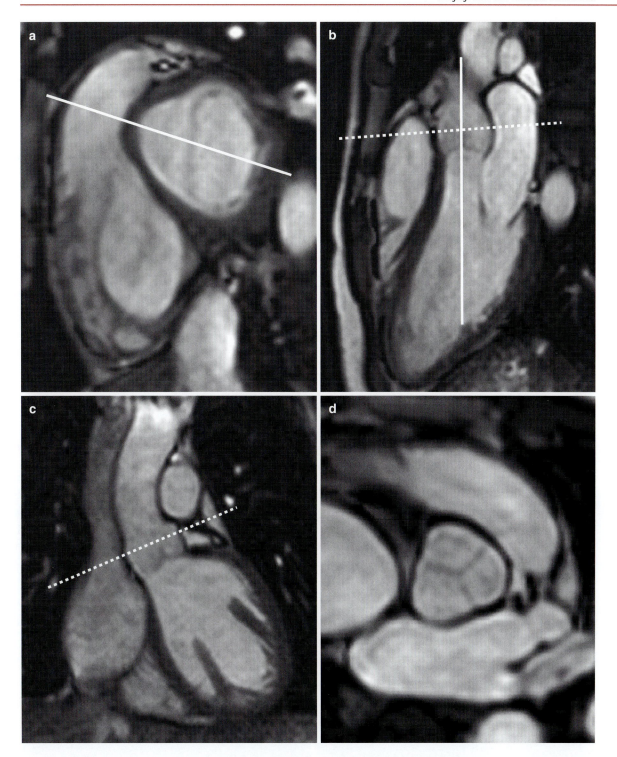

Fig. 8.1. Imaging planes can be aligned from the basal SA slice (**a**). The LV inflow (mitral valve)/outflow (aortic valve) view (**b**) acquired with a plane passing across mid-point Ao and mitral valves on the basal SA slice. A perpendicular cross-cut of the LVOT produces image (**c**). Alignment of the aortic valve plane (**d**) for aortic flow assessment from the LV inflow/ outflow (**b**) and the left ventricular outflow tract (LVOT) (**c**) views (*dotted lines*). The imaging plane should be placed just above the aortic valve, yet just below the origin of the coronary artery origins

9 Imaging Planes-Right Ventricular Outflow Tract

RVOT planned using HASTE axial images, and acquired using b-SSFP.

Pulmonary valve plane used for through-plane PA flow, and valve morphology.

These figures illustrate the process with normal anatomy. The same principles are used for patients with any ventricular arrangement.

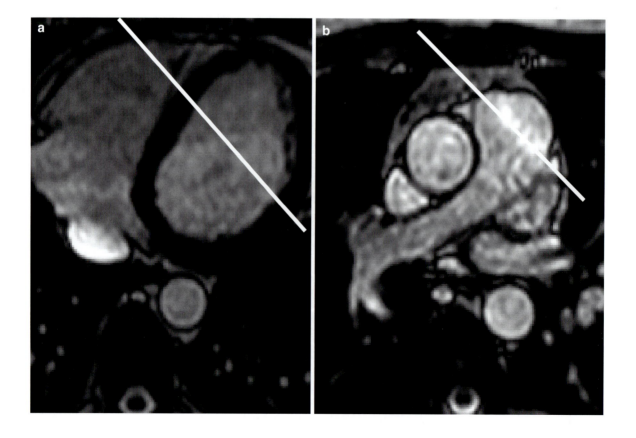

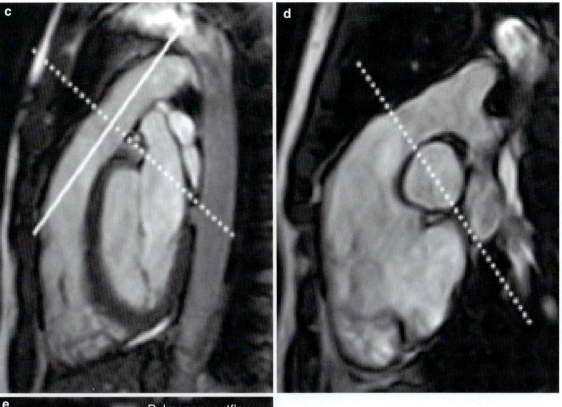

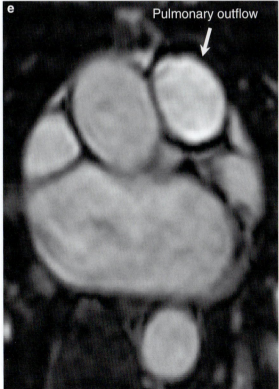

Pulmonary outflow

Fig. 9.1. Alignment of the pulmonary valve plane (**e**) for pulmonary flow assessment from two perpendicular right ventricular outflow tract (RVOT) (**c**, **d**) views (*dotted lines*). The imaging plane should be placed just above the pulmonary valve. The first RVOT view is prescribed from an oblique plane through the main pulmonary artery and RV on a set of axial images (**a**, **b**). The second RVOT plane is prescribed perpendicular to the first RVOT view (complete line on (**c**))

10a Imaging Planes-Branch PAs

The branch PAs (RPA and LPA) do not lie in the same axial plane (LPA is slightly superior to the RPA).

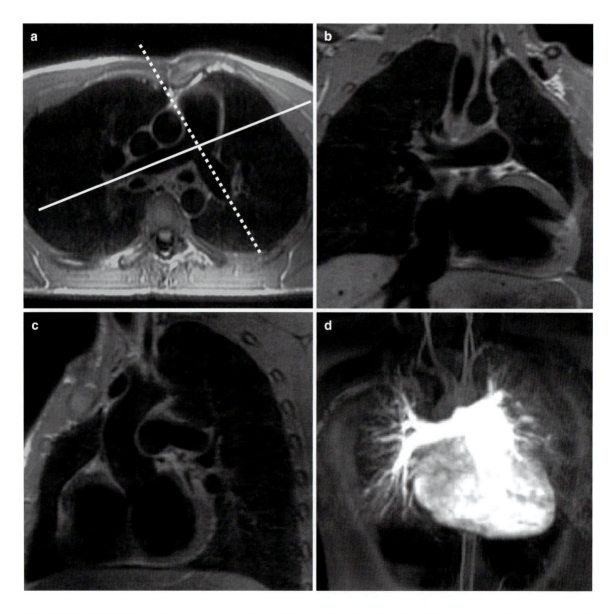

Fig. 10.1 (a-d). Both arteries can be shown in an oblique axial plane (**a**). An oblique coronal plane can be used to show the RPA (**b**). An oblique sagittal plane used to show the LPA (**c**). PA MRA shown in (**d**).

10b   Imaging Planes-Thoracic Aorta

The thoracic aorta has a complex morphology, which does not lie in a single saggital or coronal plane.

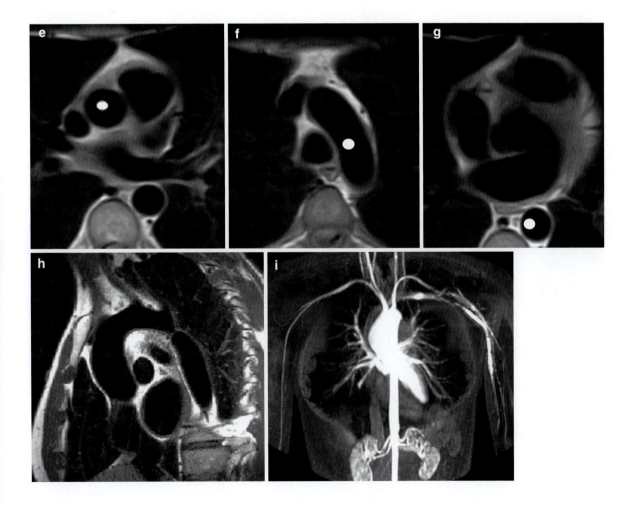

Fig. 10.1 (e -i). Alignment of the thoracic aorta using a 3-point plan. Points placed on "black-blood" axial images: (**e**) ascending aorta, (**f**) aortic arch, and (**g**) proximal descending aorta. The in-plane image of the thoracic aorta in (**h**) shows a tight aortic coarctation membrane. Aortic MRA shown in (**i**)

11a Imaging Planes-Tricuspid Valve

The imaging plane should be placed just within the RV.

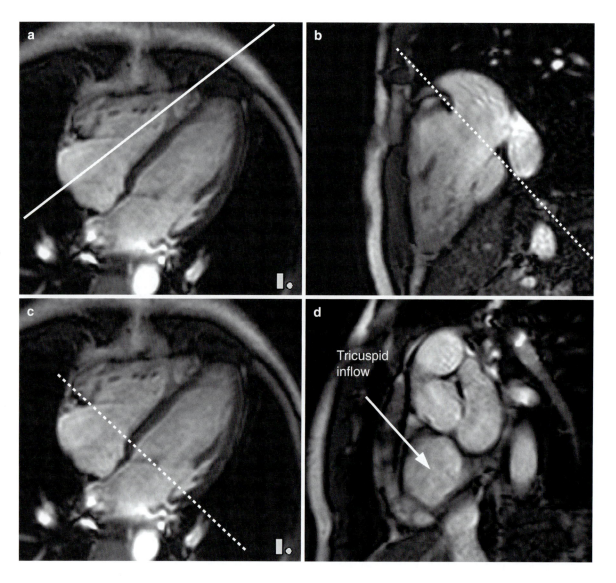

Fig. 11.1. Alignment of the tricuspid valve plane (**d**) for RV inflow assessment from the RV VLA (**b**) and the 4-chamber planes (**a, c**)

11b   Imaging Planes-Mitral Valve

The imaging plane should be placed just within the LV.

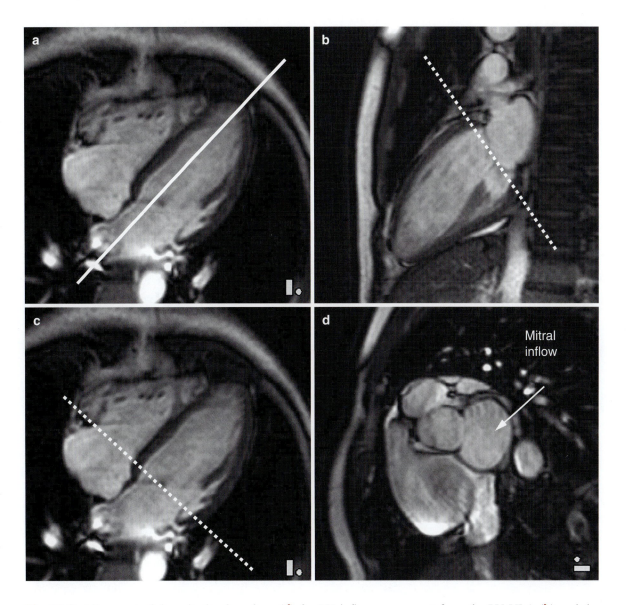

Fig. 11.2. Alignment of the mitral valve plane (**d**) for LV inflow assessment from the LV VLA (**b**) and the 4-chamber planes (**a**, **c**)

12   Imaging Planes-Coronary Arteries

MR coronary angiography is performed from alignment of a narrow 3D volume along the length of each vessel.

RCA plane is aligned off axial images using a 3-point-plane scan – RCA ostium, RCA midpoint in anterior AV-groove and (distally) inferior portion of the RCA as it passes towards the crux.

LCA tree is derived from two scans aligned using three point-plane scans facilitating visualisation of longer segments of LCA tree + branches.

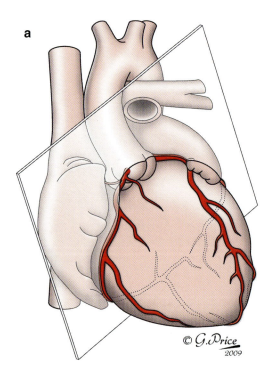

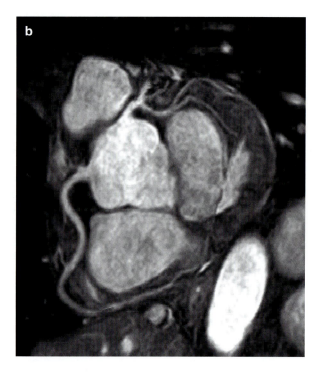

Fig. 12.1. Right coronary artery (**a**) schematic angiographic representation (**b**) 3D-whole heart image

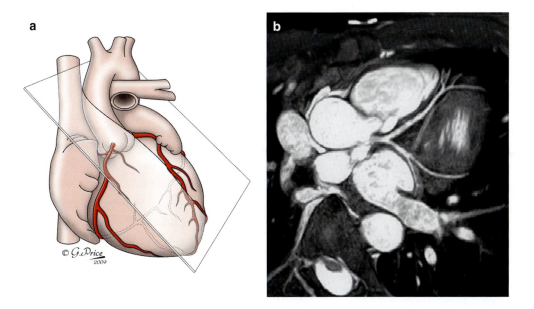

Fig. 12.2. Left main stem, LAD and circumflex arteries "tangential view" (**a**) schematic angiographic representation (**b**) 3D-whole heart image

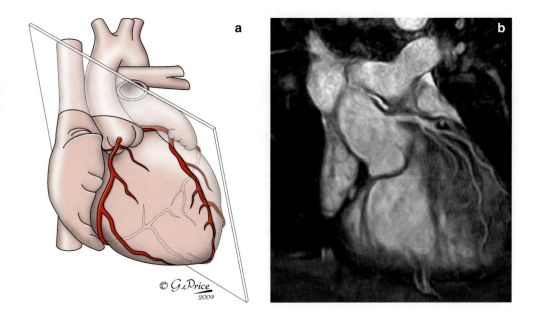

Fig. 12.3. Left main stem and LAD "perpendicular" view (**a**) schematic angiographic representation (**b**) 3D-whole heart image

13   Atrial Septal Defect

Assess defect diameter & margin size – suitability for device anchorage.

Quantify right heart volume and function – evaluate volume overload.

Quantify the shunt (Qp/Qs) – Note: PA flow velocity may be high due to increased flow volume

Look for sinus venosus defect (assess for PAPVD – right upper vein).

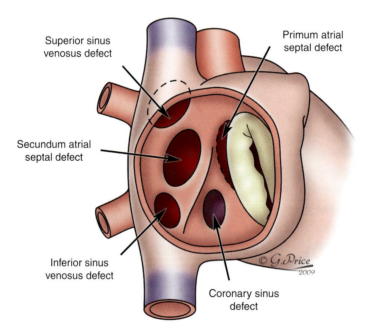

Fig. 13.1. Schematic drawing showing the various positions of the holes that permit interatrial shunting

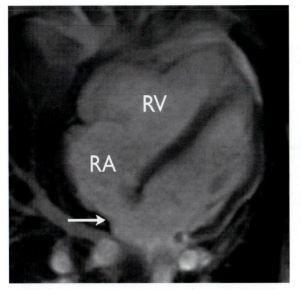

Fig. 13.2. b-SSFP image. 4-Ch view showing a large secundum ASD with posterior extension. The absence of a posterior rim (*arrow*) precludes insertion of an ASD closure device. Note the dilated right atrium, and right ventricle, and flattened interventricular septum

Fig. 13.3. Through-plane phase-encoded velocity flow map demonstrating significant flow through an ASD (*arrow*). Insert shows the imaging plane from which the flow image was acquired

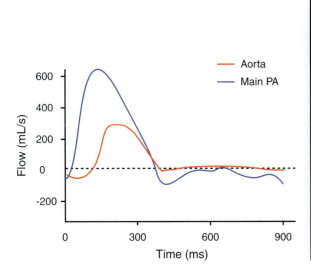

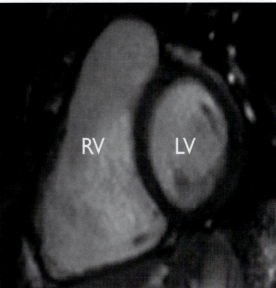

Fig. 13.4. Plot of instantaneous flow (measured by velocity-encoded phase contrast MRI) as a function of time showing a left to right shunt through an ASD. Note greater pulmonary blood flow

Fig. 13.5. b-SSFP image. SA-view showing a severely dilated right ventricle

14   Sinus Venosus Defect

Echo diagnosis can be difficult due to the posterior location of the defect.

Assess the site and size of the defect.

Delineate associated anomalous connection of the right upper pulmonary vein to the base of the superior vena cava (PAPVD).

Document the course (drainage) of all pulmonary veins.

Quantify right heart volume and function – evaluate volume overload.

Quantify the shunt (Qp/Qs).

Post op – look for SVC or redirected pulmonary vein obstruction.

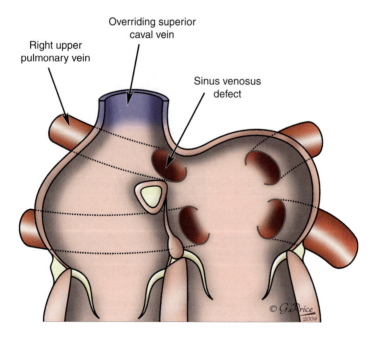

Right upper pulmonary vein

Overriding superior caval vein

Sinus venosus defect

Fig. 14.1. Schematic drawing of superior sinus venous defect. Note the high position of the defect in the atrial septum. The right upper pulmonary vein drains into the base of the defect resulting in anomalous drainage despite a usual anatomical position of the vein itself

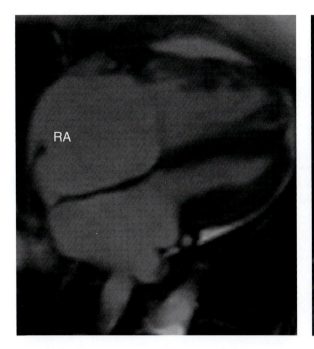

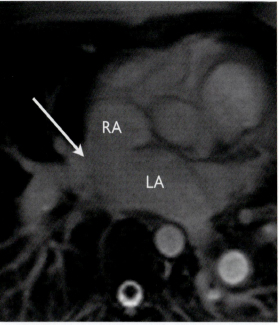

Fig. 14.2. b-SSFP image. 4-Ch view in systole, show-ing a severely dilated RA. This finding should prompt interrogation of the posterior superior atrial septum for a sinus venosus defect

Fig. 14.3. b-SSFP image. Axial view showing a sinus venosus defect in the posterior superior atrial septum. Note the PAPVD, with the right upper, and right mid-dle pulmonary veins straddling the deficient atrial sep-tum (*arrow*)

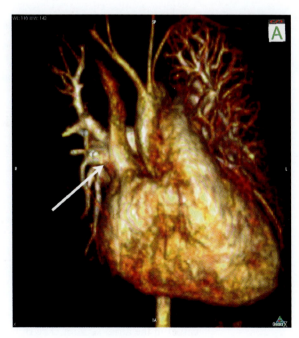

Fig. 14.4. Volume-rendered 3D reconstruction from gadolinium-enhanced MR angiogram in a patient with a sinus venosus defect, and partial anomalous pulmo-nary venous connections. The right upper and right middle pulmonary veins drain into the SVC (*arrow*). Note that the right pulmonary arterial tree has been removed for improved venous visualisation

15   Atrioventricular Septal Defect

Assess ventricular balance. Unequal commitment of common valve to ventricles may affect suitability for bi-ventricular repair.

Assess valve structure in terms of potential for repair.

Look for chordal attachments crossing VSD (*better seen on echo*) as it may affect surgical strategy.

Look for associated abnormalities – isomerism or great vessel disorders.

Quantify ventricular volume and function – evaluate volume overload.

Quantify the shunt (Qp/Qs).

Evaluate degree of AV valve regurgitation.

Post op – residual shunt, degree AV valve regurgitation or stenosis, LVOT obstruction, ventricular size & function

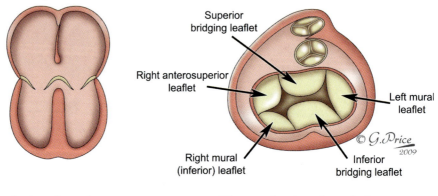

4-chamber view   Short axis view from below

Fig. 15.1. Schematic drawing of atrioventricular septal defect. Orthogonal views of common valve

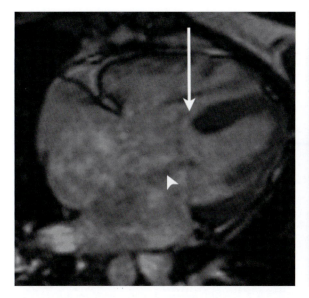

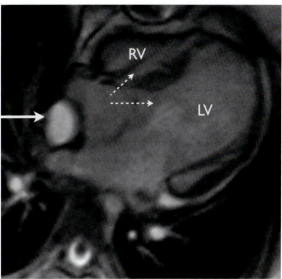

Fig. 15.2. b-SSFP image. 4-Ch view showing a balanced complete AVSD. There are large atrial and ventricular components. Note that the SB leaflet is largely contained within the LV with chordal attachment to the septal crest (Rastelli Type A) (*arrow*). Also note the moderate left AV valve regurgitation (*arrowhead*)

Fig. 15.3. b-SSFP image. 4-Ch view showing an unbalanced complete AVSD. Note that 50% of the right AV valve is committed to the left ventricle, and the right ventricle is hypoplastic. The *dotted line* shows the direction of flow through the tricuspid valve to both ventricles. *Arrow* denotes the lateral tunnel part of this patient's TCPC (Fontan) circulation

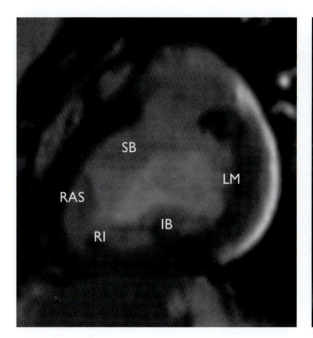

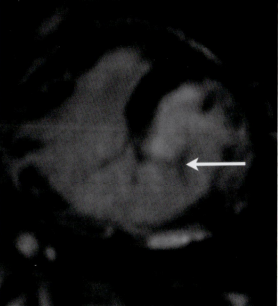

Fig. 15.4. b-SSFP image. Valve view showing a complete AVSD in a patient with right isomerism, and double outlet right ventricle. Valve leaflets as in Fig. 15.1

Fig. 15.5. b-SSFP image. Valve view showing a balanced partial AVSD. A tongue of tissue joins SB and IB, making left AV valve trileaflet (*arrow*), with the right AV valve having four leaflets

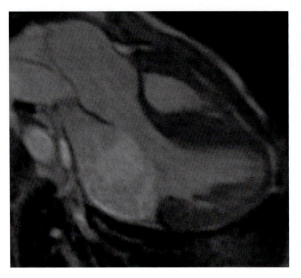

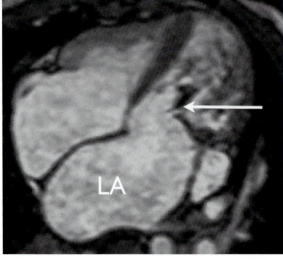

Fig. 15.6. b-SSFP image. LVOT view in a patient with a partial AVSD. Due to the common AV valve, the aorta has been displaced anteriorly, with subsequent elongation of the LVOT – the so-called "goose-neck" deformity. This can lead to outflow tract obstruction

Fig. 15.7. b-SSFP image. 4- Ch view showing a repair of balanced complete AVSD. The ventricular septum is intact, however there is now a functional narrowing of the left AV valve, with diastolic flow acceleration into the LV (*arrow*). Note the moderately dilated LA

Notes

16   Ventricular Septal Defect

Assess position and size of defects – possibly multiple defects.

Quantify the shunt (Qp/Qs).

The shunt will be proportional to the size of the defect, and the SVR:PVR ratio.

Note: Unlike an ASD, LV stroke volume contributes to the PA forward flow during left to right shunting.

Quantify ventricular volume and function – evaluate volume overload.

Assess for the presence of aortic regurgitation observed with perimembranous defects.

Look for associated abnormalities – aortic arch anomalies, aortic coarctation, pulmonary stenosis.

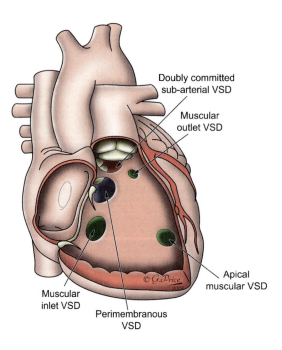

Fig. 16.1. Schematic drawing showing the categorization used for differentiation of the various types of ventricular septal defect. Viewed from a right ventricular aspect

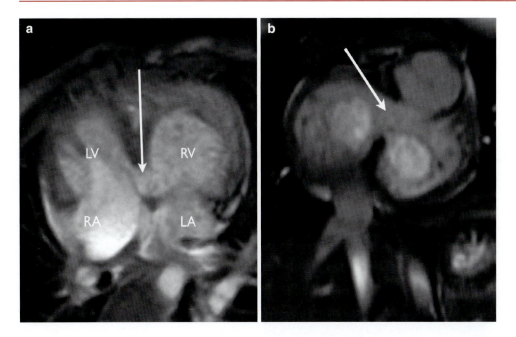

Fig. 16.2. b-SSFP images of an inlet VSD (*arrow*) in a patient with congenitally corrected transposition of the great arteries (**a**) 4-Ch and (**b**) SA views

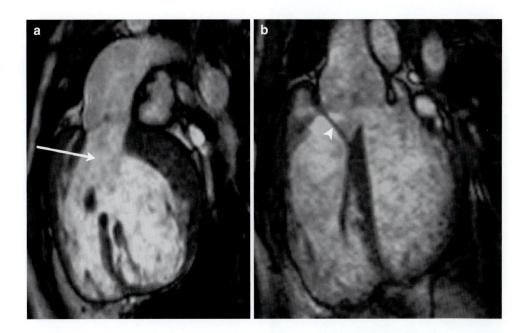

Fig. 16.3. b-SSFP images of a VSD (*arrow*) with over-riding aorta in a patient with Tetralogy of Fallot (coronal oblique view (**a**, **b**) coronal oblique view following correction with VSD patch (*arrowhead*)

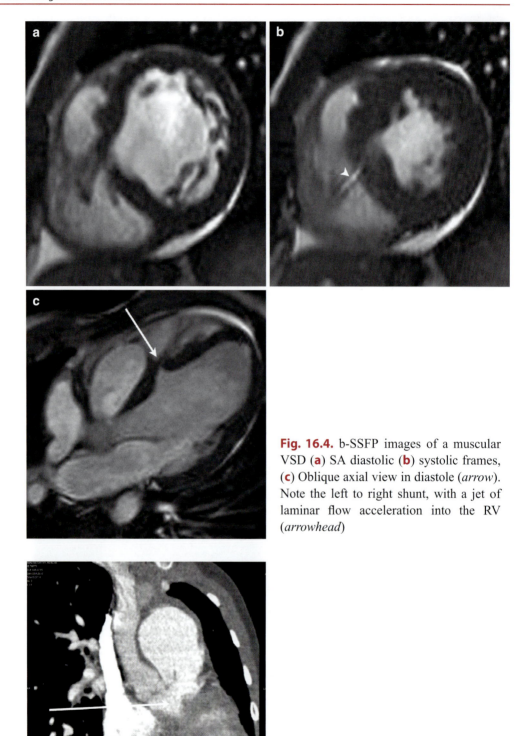

Fig. 16.4. b-SSFP images of a muscular VSD (**a**) SA diastolic (**b**) systolic frames, (**c**) Oblique axial view in diastole (*arrow*). Note the left to right shunt, with a jet of laminar flow acceleration into the RV (*arrowhead*)

Fig. 16.5. Coronal oblique MPR CT image of a doubly committed VSD (*arrow*)

Simple shunt quantification

Suspect a shunt if there is
Asymmetric atrial or ventricular dilatation
Dilatation of the main and branch pulmonary arteries

Always assess
Ventricular stroke volumes
Aortic and pulmonary flow volumes

Note: The presence of AV valve regurgitation can confound the simple guides below

VSD shunt	Usual
Pure Left to right Qp > Qs	RVSV = Ao FF
	LVSV = Pulm FF
	Pulm FF > Ao FF
	LVSV > RVSV

VSD shunt	RV high pressure
Pure Right to left Qp < Qs	RVSV = Ao FF
	LVSV = Pulm FF
	Ao FF > Pulm FF
	RVSV > LVSV

ASD shunt	Usual
Pure Left to right Qp > Qs	RVSV = Pulm FF
	LVSV = Ao FF
	Pulm FF > Ao FF
	RVSV > LVSV

ASD shunt	RV low compliance
Pure Right to left Qp < Qs	RVSV = Pulm FF
	LVSV = Ao FF
	Ao FF > Pulm FF
	LVSV > RVSV

Through-plane flow volume assessment:
- Phase-contrast, through-plane flow mapping.
- Use high spatial and temporal resolution sequences (free-breathing)
- Place slice perpendicular to both orthogonal long axis views through the great vessel.
- Place slice in an area of laminar flow, distal to semi-lunar valve tips. Proximal to the first aortic or pulmonary artery branches.

Ventricular volume assessment:
- b-SSFP images with temporal resolution at least 50 ms.
- Use short axis or horizonal long axis slices, with no gap.
- A slice-positioning tool improves accuracy of segmentation for basal slices.
- Exclude major trabeculae from blood pool.
- Manual tracing is currently the most precise processing method for RVSV

18   Aortic Valve Incompetence

Assess valve leaflet structure (e.g. bicuspid valve) and mechanism of regurgitation – coaptation defect vs. prolapse

Evaluate aortic root dilation.

Visualise regurgitant jet using orthogonal planes.

Quantify regurgitant fraction – grading: mild 10–20%, moderate 20–40%, severe >40%.

Quantify LV volumes and systolic function.

Look for additional pre and post-surgical causes: Marfan, dissection, infection or vegetation (if large) or abscess.

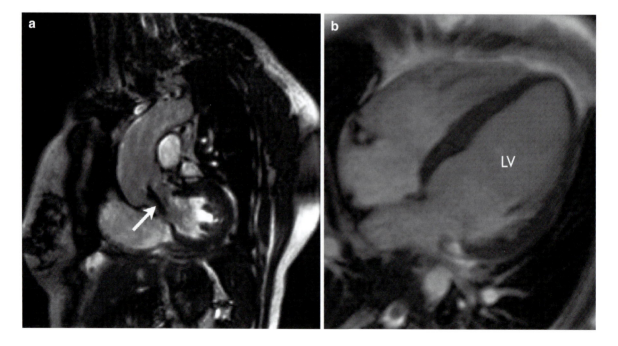

Fig. 18.1. (a) b-SSFP image oblique coronal view, showing narrow jet of moderate aortic regurgitation. **(b)** b-SSFP images showing a 4-Ch view of a dilated left ventricle in a patient with aortic regurgitation

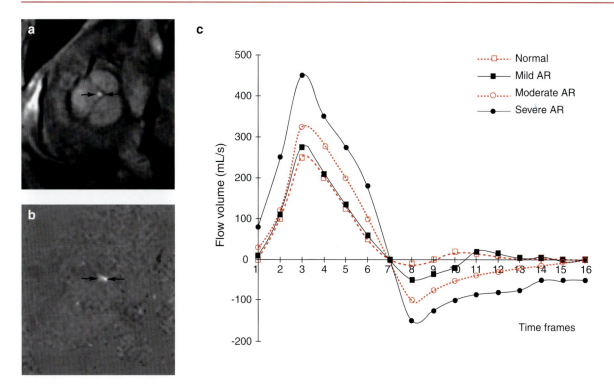

Fig. 18.2. Aortic regurgitation phase contrast velocity mapping, (**a**) magnitude image aortic valve, (**b**) phase contrast image above the aortic valve in early diastole showing a narrow jet of regurgitation (high signal). (**c**) Aortic regurgitation flow vs. time plot for the ascending aorta for different grades of regurgitation, compared to a normal flow curve

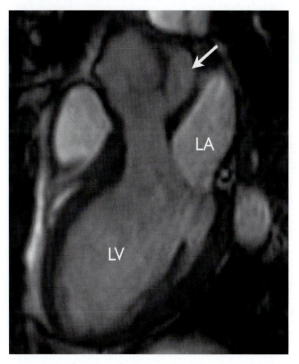

Fig. 18.3. b-SSFP left ventricular inflow/outflow view, in a patient who has undergone the Ross procedure, showing a large aortic root abscess extending between the pulmonary autograft, and left atrium

19   Coarctation of the Aorta

Describe the location and degree of the stenotic region (often focal)/length of coarctation segment.

Look for arch involvement and post stenotic dilatation.

Assess aortic root and valve – often bicuspid.

Delineate collateral vessels.

Describe head and neck vessel anatomy in relation to coarctation.

Assess ventricular function, volumes and LV mass (may be increased 2° LVOTO or hypertension).

Measure peak CoA velocity, look for diastolic prolongation of forward flow.

Look for associated anomalies – sub-aortic VSD, berry aneurysms, renal artery stenosis.

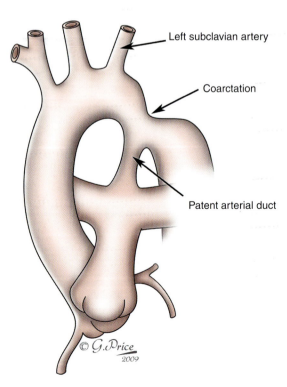

Left subclavian artery

Coarctation

Patent arterial duct

© G.Price 2009

Fig. 19.1. Schematic drawing of coarctation distal to left subclavian artery. Note site of coarctation opposite the patent arterial duct and distal to the left subclavian artery

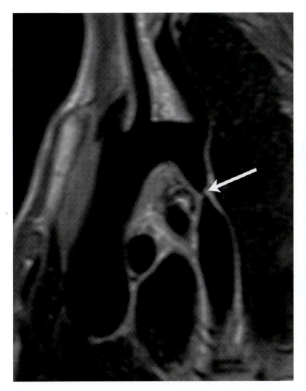

Fig. 19.2. BB TSE oblique sagittal image through the aorta showing a tight discrete coarctation (*arrow*)

Fig. 19.3. Volume rendered 3D reconstruction of a CE-MRA showing a tight coarctation (*arrowhead*), and multiple enlarged collateral vessels

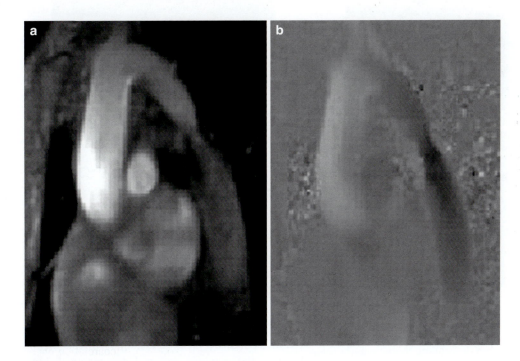

Fig. 19.4. Magnitude (**a**), and phase contrast image (**b**) of a moderate coarctation

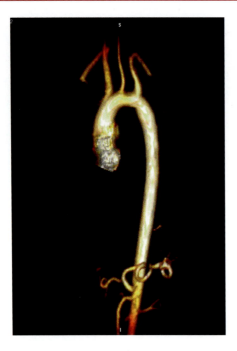

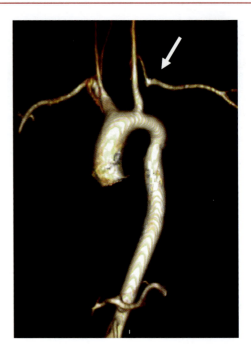

Fig. 19.5. Volume rendered 3D reconstruction of a CE-MRA showing a good coarctation repair following end-to-end anastamosis. Note Roman arch morphology

Fig. 19.6. Volume rendered 3D reconstruction of a CE-MRA showing a subclavian flap repair of a coarctation. Note the LSA filling via vertebral collaterals (*arrow*), and the persistent hypoplasia of the transverse arch (*arrowhead*)

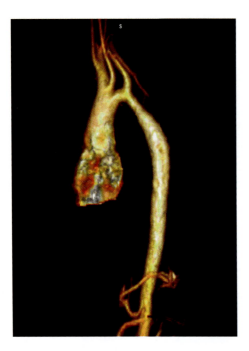

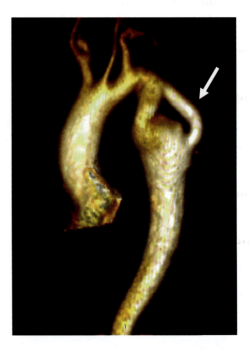

Fig. 19.7. Volume rendered 3D reconstruction of a CE-MRA showing moderate to severe residual narrowing of the proximal descending thoracic aorta following patch aortoplasty. Note dilated aortic root due to bicuspid aortopathy and Gothic arch morphology

Fig. 19.8. Volume rendered 3D reconstruction of a CE-MRA showing an extra-anatomic conduit (*arrow*) between the proximal and mid descending thoracic aorta

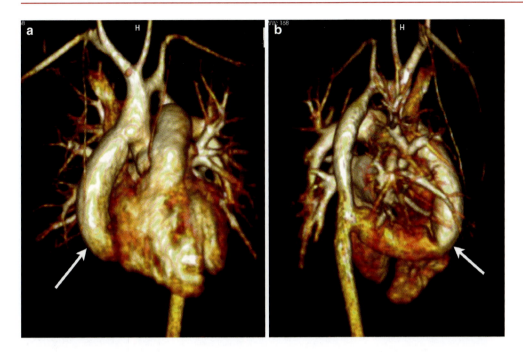

Fig. 19.9. Long-segment severe narrowing of the descending thoracic aorta with extra-anatomic conduit (*arrow*) connecting the ascending and distal descending aorta. (**a**) anterior, and (**b**) posterior views from a volume rendered 3D reconstruction of a CE-MRA

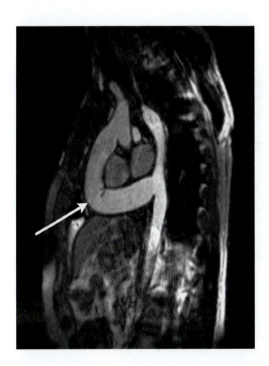

Fig. 19.10. 3D b-SSFP sagittal image.showing a long-segment severe narrowing of the descending thoracic aorta with extra-anatomic conduit (*arrow*) connecting the ascending and distal descending aorta

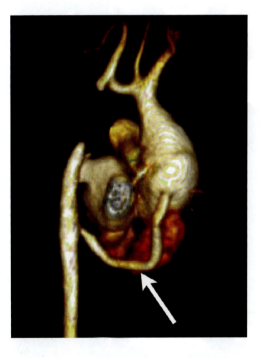

Fig. 19.11. Volume rendered 3D reconstruction of a CE-MRA showing interruption of the proximal descending thoracic aorta with extra-anatomic conduit (*arrow*) connecting the ascending and distal descending aorta

21   Interrupted Aortic Arch

Describe the site of interruption and relation to head + neck vessels.

Look for any arch hypoplasia.

Measure aortic cross-sectional area (before, and after interruption).

Measure size of "interruption gap" to aid surgical planning.

Look for associated anomalies – VSD with posterior deviation of outlet septum producing LVOT obstruction, TGA, truncus arteriosus.

Also look for: presence of thymus (as absence supports associated risk of 22q11 deletion).

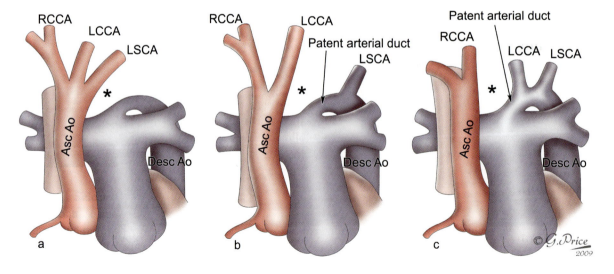

Fig. 21.1. Schematic drawing of Interruption of the aorta at differing sites. (**a**) Interruption distal to left subclavian artery (Type A). (**b**) Between left common carotid artery and left subclavian artery (Type B) (**c**) between right sub-clavian artery and left common carotid artery (Type C). Note - Interruption gap is represented by *. AscAo = ascending aorta, RCCA = right common carotid artery, LCCA=left common carotid artery, LSCA = left subclavian artery, DescAo = descending aorta

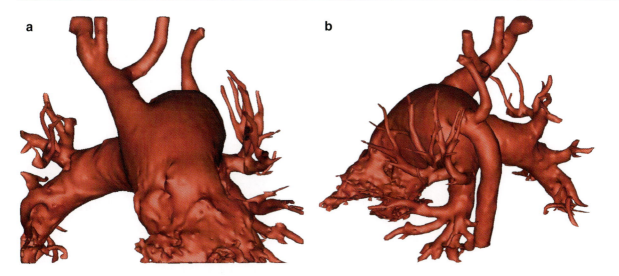

Fig. 21.2. Volume rendered contrast enhanced CT images of a patient with a Type B interruption of the aortic arch and Truncus arteriosus, (**a**) anterior, and (**b**) posterior oblique views

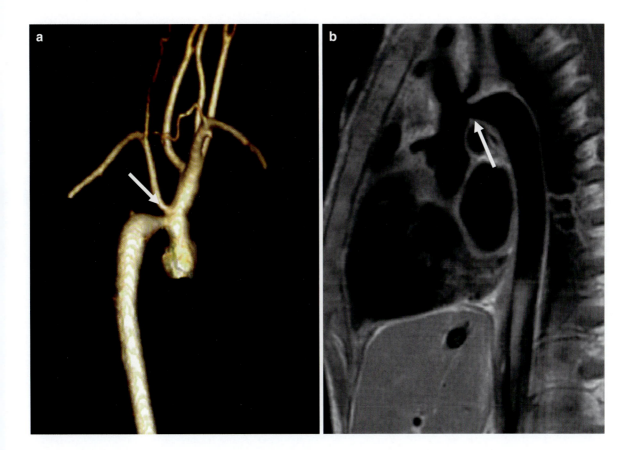

Fig. 21.3. Selected images of a corrected type A interruption of the aortic arch, with moderate narrowing at the site of end to side anastomosis (*arrow*). (**a**) VR 3D reconstruction CE-MRA (viewed from the right), (**b**) BB TSE sagittal view.

22 Aortic Vascular Rings

Assess arch number & calibre

Describe branching pattern of head & neck vessels.

Describe presence & course of aberrant subclavian artery, aorta & descending aorta – is descending aorta retro-oesophageal?

Look for atretic fibrous arch/ductal ligament – not seen on MR, but presence can be implied by shape of aorta.

Check for presence of Kommeral's diverticulum.

Importance of airway assessment – recommend concomitant spiral CT angiography + dynamic contrast bronchography.

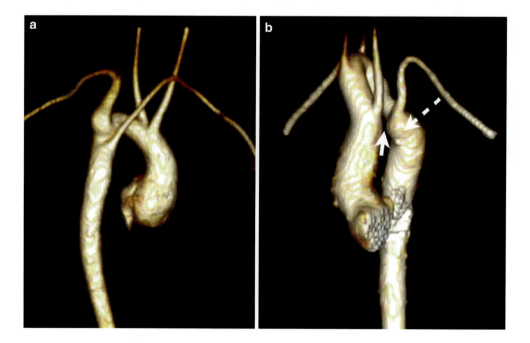

Fig. 22.1. Volume rendered 3D reconstructions from CE-MRA of the aorta showing (**a**) left aortic arch with aberrant right subclavian artery and right cervical aortic arch with aberrant left subclavian artery. (**b**) there is likely to be a fibrous band connecting the brachiocephalic artery and aberrant left subclavian artery representing an atrophied left arch (*arrow*), which is not seen. A further band may also be present between the Kommerell's diverticulum (*dashed arrow*) and left pulmonary artery

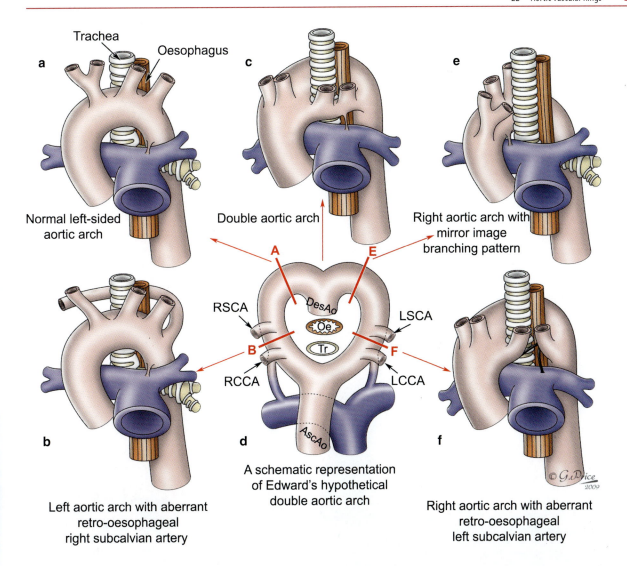

a Normal left-sided aortic arch

Trachea
Oesophagus

b Left aortic arch with aberrant retro-oesophageal right subcalvian artery

c Double aortic arch

d A schematic representation of Edward's hypothetical double aortic arch

RSCA
RCCA
LSCA
LCCA
DesAo
Oe
Tr
AscAo
A   E
B   F

e Right aortic arch with mirror image branching pattern

f Right aortic arch with aberrant retro-oesophageal left subcalvian artery

© G.Price 2009

Fig. 22.2. (d) Shows a schematic representation of Edward's hypothetical double aortic arch, showing right and left aortic arches and bilateral arterial ducts. RCCA = right common cartid artery, RSCA=right subclavian artery, LSCA=left subclavian artery, LCCA=left common carotid artery, Oe=oesophagus, Tr=trachea, DesAo=descending aorta, AscAo=ascending aorta. (**c**) shows a double aortic arch. Division of the double arch (in (**d**)) along the line A gives (**a**), a normal left-sided aortic arch. Division of the double arch along the line B gives (**b**), a left aortic arch with aberrant retro-oesophageal right subclavian artery. Division along the line E gives (**e**), a right-sided aortic arch with mirror image branching. Division along the line F, gives (**f**); an artist impression of a right arch with retro-esophageal aortic arch / aberrant left subclavian artery. The black lines in image **f** represent potential complete vascular rings of an atretic left arch (superior line) and a fibrotic left arterial duct (inferior line)

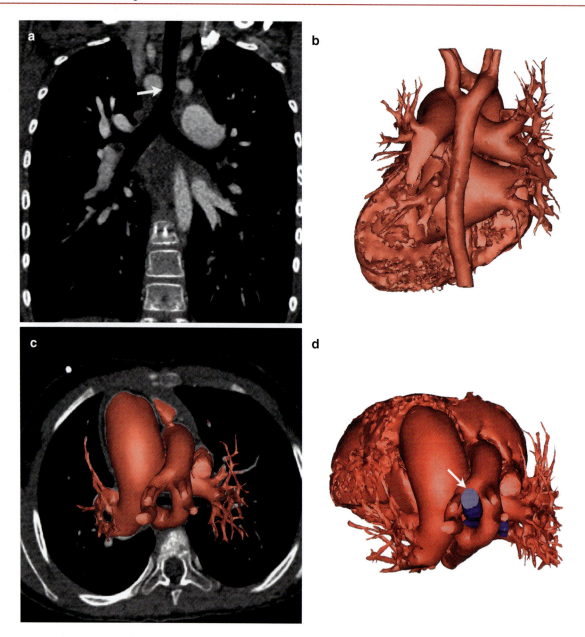

Fig. 22.3. Selected images from contrast-enhanced CT showing a double arch. (**a**) coronal MPR – note the mild side-to-side narrowing of the trachea (*arrow*) as the left and right aortic arches pass to either side (**b**, **c**) and (**d**) Volume-rendered 3D reconstructions (**b**) posterior view, (**c**) superior view superimposed onto a background of the axial CT and (**d**) superior view with volume rendering of the trachea also shown (*arrow*)

Notes

23   Left Pulmonary Artery Sling

Describe course, size and any stenosis of branch PAs.

Assess for presence of complete cartilaginous tracheal rings.

Quantify RV systolic function, volume, hypertrophy.

Quantify branch pulmonary artery flow volumes.

Branch pulmonary artery flow volumes

Post op – assess adequacy of LPA re-implantation and exclude branch PA stenosis at site of native origin in distal RPA.

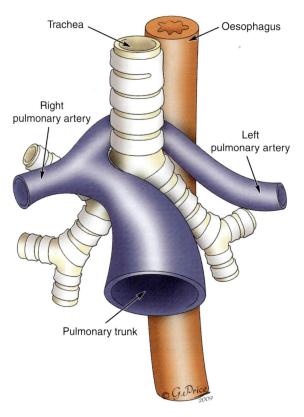

Fig. 23.1. Schematic drawing of left pulmonary artery sling

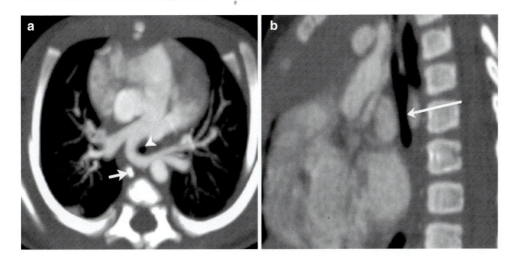

Fig. 23.2. LPA sling (**a**) axial MIP image from a post-contrast CT showing distal take-off of LPA from RPA and its subsequent retro-tracheal course. Nasogastric tube (*arrow*); trachea (*arrowhead*), (**b**) sagittal MPR CT image – note the mild narrowing of the trachea as it passes between MPA and LPA (*arrow*)

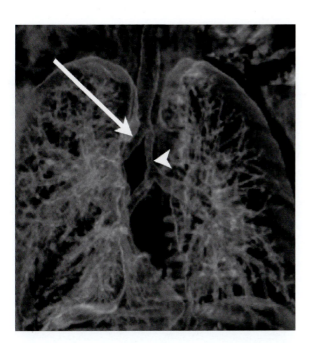

Fig. 23.3. Volume rendered 3D reconstruction from a thoracic CT, showing an accessory right upper lobe "pig" bronchus (*arrow*), and a "stove pipe" distal trachea proximal to the carina (*arrowhead*). This tracheobronchial anatomy is associated with the LPA sling

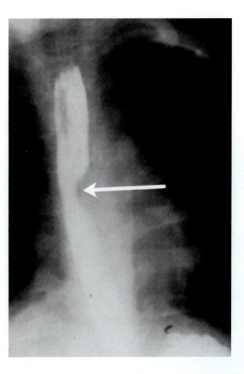

Fig. 23.4. Right anterior oblique projection from a barium swallow, showing anterior oesophageal indentation (*arrow*)

24   Marfan Syndrome

Quantify aortic arch dilatation ± dissection (often focal).

Quantify aortic regurgitation.

Assess mechanism of regurgitation.

Assess left ventricular volumes and systolic function.

Look for spine dural ectasia.

Differentiate from Loeys-Dietz syndrome – tortous head, neck and arch vessels.

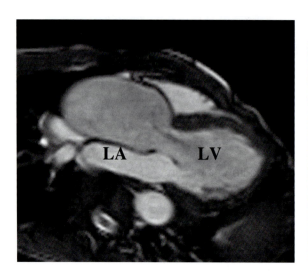

Fig. 24.1. Left ventricular outflow tract view (b-SSFP) showing dilated aortic root and aortic valve regurgitation

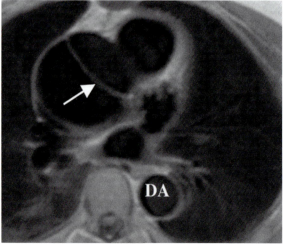

Fig. 24.2. Axial BB TSE image showing dilated aortic root with dissection flap (*arrow*)

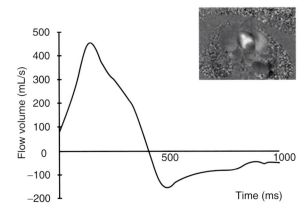

Fig. 24.3. Flow curve derived from phase contrast image (*inset*) demonstrating significant aortic valve regurgitation (fraction 30%)

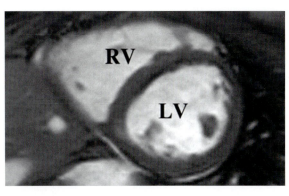

Fig. 24.4. b-SSFP SA image showing left ventricular dilatation

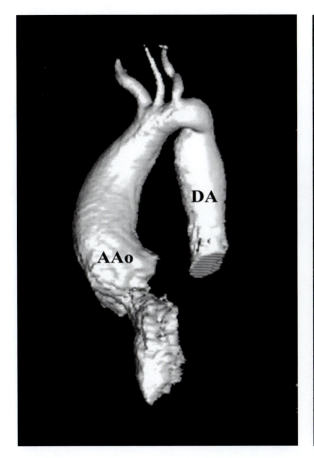

Fig. 24.5. 3D reconstruction CE-MRA of the aortic arch showing a dilated aortic root and pseudo-coarctation

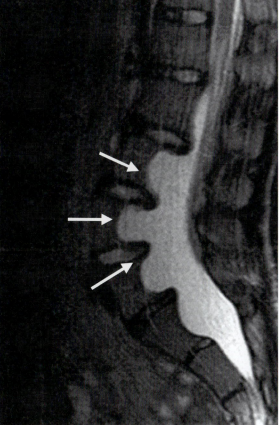

Fig. 24.6. Sagittal section through the spinal cord (T2-weighted) showing dural ectasia (*arrows*)

25 Williams Syndrome

Assess supravalvar aortic stenosis.

Look for arch hypoplasia and coarctation.

Identify any branch and peripheral pulmonary artery stenosis.

Identify any other arterial stenoses: coronary, head & neck vessels, renal arteries.

Identify degree of arterial wall thickening in all vessels.

Quantify gradient across aortic stenosis (peak velocity) & branch PAs.

Assess ventricular function, volumes and mass.

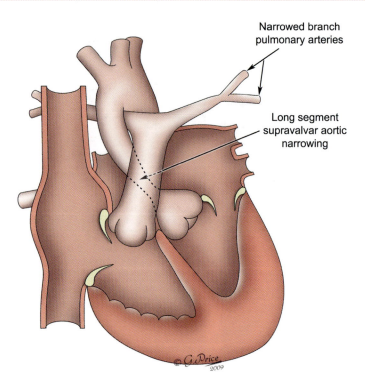

Fig. 25.1. Schematic drawing of Williams syndrome

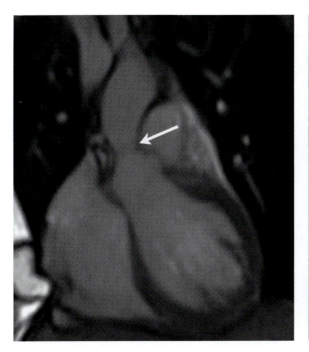

Fig. 25.2. b-SSFP aortic outflow image showing supra-valvar aortic stenosis (*arrow*)

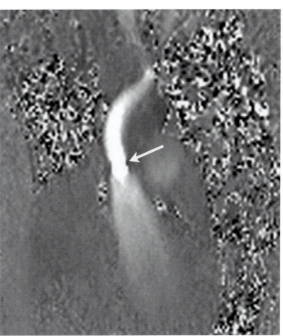

Fig. 25.3. In-plane phase contrast image showing flow acceleration (*arrow*) originating at a supra-valvar level extending into the aortic arch

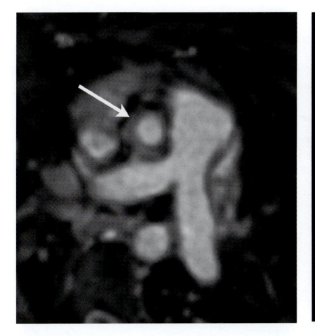

Fig. 25.4. 3D b-SSFP axial image showing thickening of the aortic wall (*arrow*) at the level of the supra-valvar narrowing

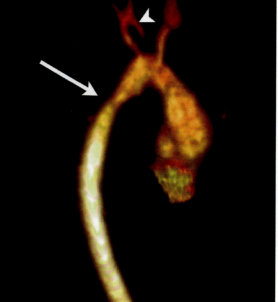

Fig. 25.5. Volume rendered 3D CE-MRA. The supra-valvar narrowing has been repaired with a pericardial patch, but there is residual narrowing of the aortic arch and proximal descending thoracic aorta (*arrow*). Note also that the left common carotid artery is occluded, and has a side-to-side anastomosis with the left subclavian artery (*arrowhead*)

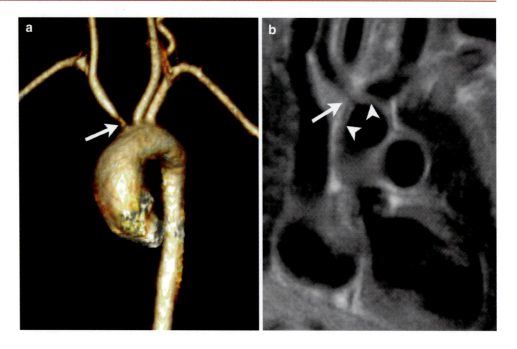

Fig. 25.6. Proximal narrowing of the brachiocephalic artery (*arrow*) in a patient with Williams syndrome, (**a**) volume rendered 3D gadolinium enhanced MRA and (**b**) BB TSE – note the arterial wall thickening (*arrowheads*) at the site of narrowing

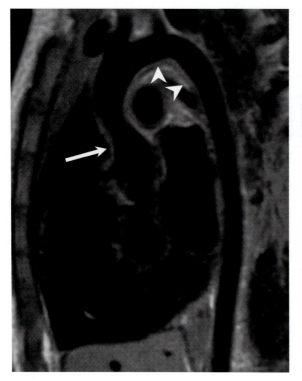

Fig. 25.7. BB TSE showing supravalvar aortic stenosis (*arrow*), aortic wall thickening (*arrowheads*), and long-segment narrowing of the descending aorta

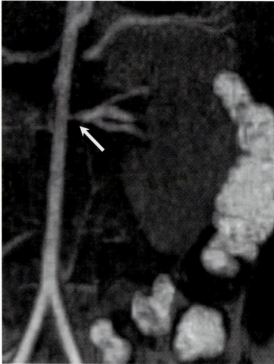

Fig. 25.8. CE MRA showing proximal left renal artery stenosis (*arrow*)

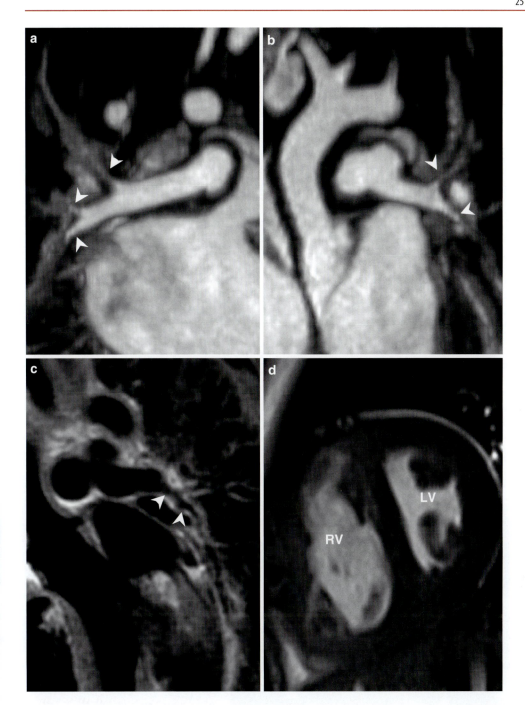

Fig. 25.9. Selected images showing severe peripheral branch pulmonary stenoses (*arrowheads*) (**a**, **b**) 3D b-SSFP images, (**c**) BB TSE, and (**d**) SA b-SSFP image – note the hypertrophy of the left and right ventricles, and systolic septal flattening in a patient with coexistent severe supravalvar aortic narrowing

26 Mitral Stenosis

Assess valvar area (planimetry).

Quantify peak velocity and mean gradient (below level of MV).

Quantify mitral regurgitation.

Assess LV volumes, systolic function.

Evaluate LA dilatation.

Assess valve structure and mechanism of stenosis.

Identify signs of pulmonary hypertension – RV hypertrophy, PA dilatation.

Look for associated anomalies – myxoma, atrial thombi, other cardiac valves (rheumatic disease).

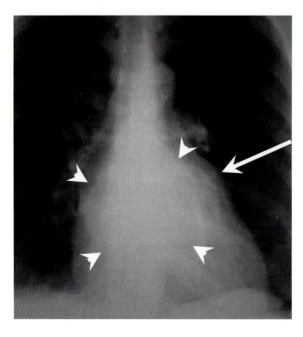

Fig. 26.1. Chest radiograph showing isolated left atrial dilatation – double shadow (*arrowheads*), splaying of the carina, prominent left atrial appendage (*arrow*), consistent with mixed mitral valve disease. Note that lack of LV dilatation shows this to be isolated mitral stenosis

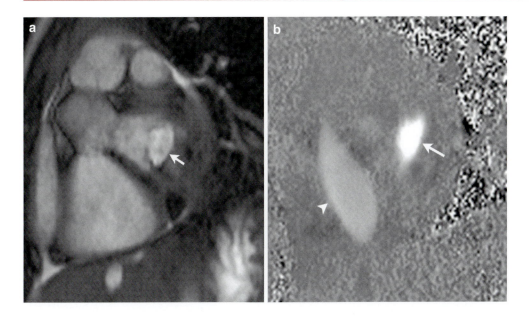

Fig. 26.2. (**a**) b-SSFP basal short axis image in mid-diastole, showing a small mitral valve orifice (*arrow*). (**b**) Through-plane phase-contrast image at the level of the atrioventicular valves. Note the much higher signal (reflecting higher velocity), and smaller area of the mitral valve flow (*arrow*), compared to the lower velocity tricuspid inflow (*arrowhead*)

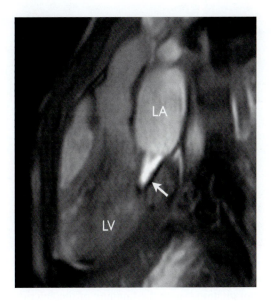

Fig. 26.3. b-SSFP image in mid-diastole-left ventricle inflow/outflow view. Flow acceleration is seen across the mitral valve (*arrow*)

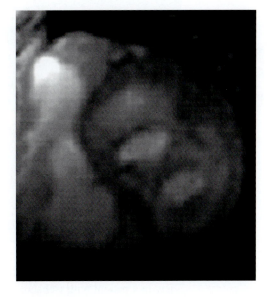

Fig. 26.4. b-SSFP basal SA view of a rare double mitral valve orifice

27   Mitral Regurgitation

Describe mechanism of regurgitation – dysplastic or prolapsing valve, papillary dysfunction, rheumatic change, LV dilation.

Visualise regurgitant jet (long axis).

Calculate regurgitation fraction – direct or indirect techniques (see haemodynamic calculations).

Assess other valves.

Look for evidence of endocarditis, myocardial infarction (LGE), cardiomyopathy.

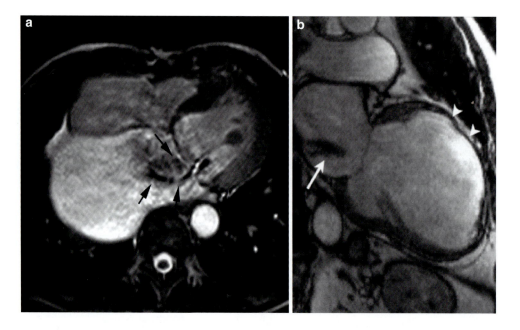

Fig. 27.1. b-SSFP images of mitral regurgitation (*arrows*). (**a**) 4-Ch, (**b**) vertical long-axis view in a patient with ischaemic mitral regurgitation – note the thinning of the anterior LV wall (*arrowheads*)

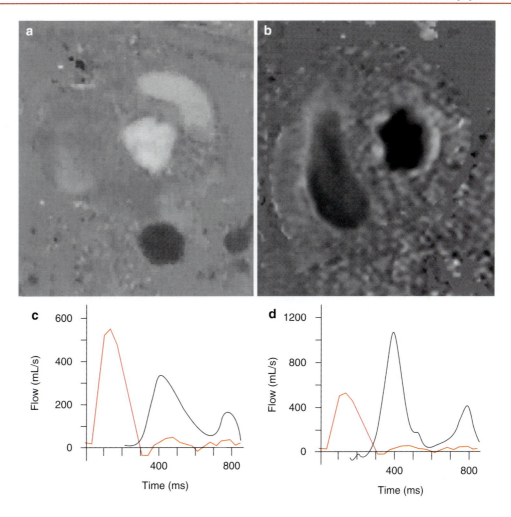

Fig. 27.2. Quantification of mitral regurgitation using phase velocity-encoded MRI to measure the difference between aortic outflow (**a**), and mitral inflow (**b**). The graphs show flow volume vs. time for mitral inflow (*black curve*), and aortic outflow (*red curve*) in a normal patient (**c**), and a patient with mitral regurgitation (**d**). The difference between the areas under the curve is the amount of regurgitation

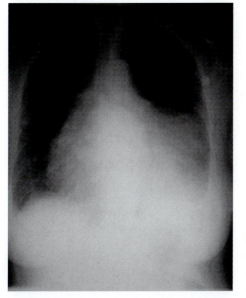

Fig. 27.3. Chest radiograph showing left atrial dilatation (see Fig 26.1), but also marked LV dilatation, consistent with mixed mitral valve disease

28 Hypertrophic Cardiomyopathy

Assess phenotypic expression – asymmetric involvement of the IVS (most common), but can also be apical and mid-ventricular.

Assess left ventricular wall thickness (measure LV myocardium in diastole on basal-, mid- and apical short axis).

Identify any LVOTO (seen in 20–30%) and describe mechanism – systolic anterior motion of MV apparatus.

Quantify LV mass, chamber size and systolic function.

Perform LGE and describe pattern of enhancement if present.

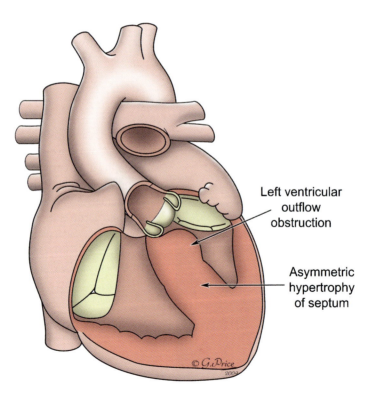

Left ventricular outflow obstruction

Asymmetric hypertrophy of septum

Fig. 28.1. Schematic drawing of hypertrophic cardiomyopathy (HOCM). Note the asymmetric hypertrophy of the interventricular septum which produces a substrate for left ventricular outflow obstruction

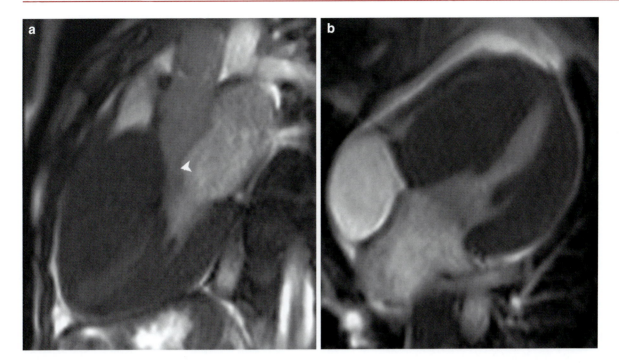

Fig. 28.2. Severe hypertrophic obstructive cardiomyopathy b-SSFP images (**a**) Left ventricular inflow/outflow view showing LVOT obstruction, and systolic anterior motion of the mitral valve (*arrowhead*), as abnormal flow pushes the mitral valve into the outflow tract. (**b**) Four chamber view

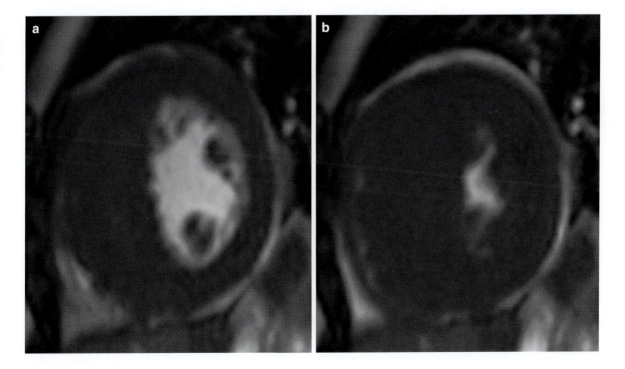

Fig. 28.3. Severe hypertrophic obstructive cardiomyopathy balanced-SSFP images (**a**) short axis view diastole, (**b**) short axis view systole

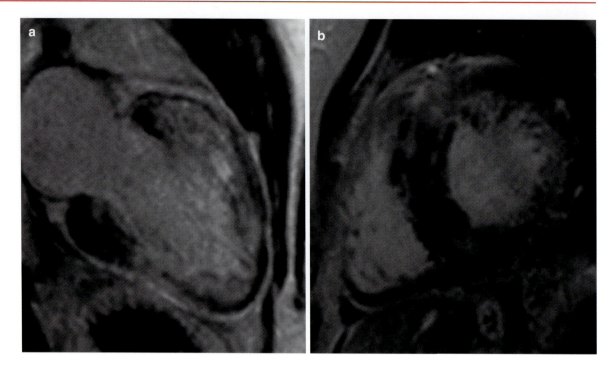

Fig. 28.4. CE inversion recovery MRI images showing extensive patchy enhancement of the thickened myocardium (**a**) VLAview of the left ventricle, (**b**) SA view

Notes

29   Dilated Cardiomypathy

Quantify LV and RV volumes, mass and function.

Look for segmental abnormality, – suggesting ischaemic pathology or if in the RV anterior wall ARVC.

Perform gadolinium enhancement scanning – early scans show thrombus.

Describe pattern of LGE: Subendocardial or segmental – ischaemic scarring, mid-myocardial – idiopathic DCM (4Ch & VLA views), patchy mid-myocardial or epicardial – possibly myocarditis (viral, inflammatory, sarcoidosis).

Look for ALCAPA as an ischaemic cause of LV dilation.

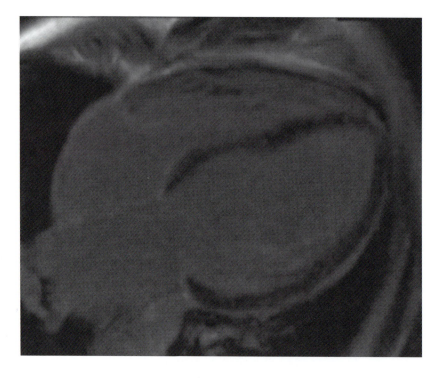

Fig. 29.1. CE-IR MRI 4-Ch view in a patient with idiopathic dilated cardiomyopathy shows no evidence of late gadolinium enhancement

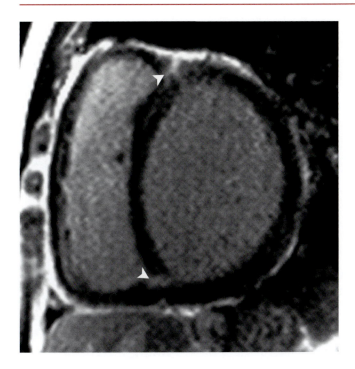

Fig. 29.2. CE-IR MRI images. SA view in a patient with idiopathic dilated cardiomyopathy shows late gadolinium enhancement (increased signal) in the region of the inferior RV insertion point (*arrowheads*)

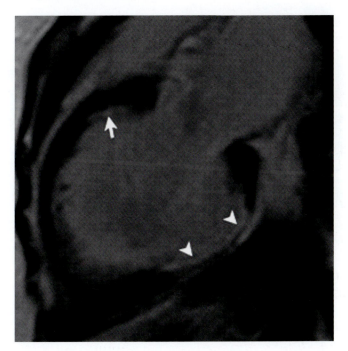

Fig. 29.3. CE-IR MRI vertical long axis image in a patient with ischaemic dilated cardiomyopathy. There is evidence of late gadolinium enhancement, with full thickness (high signal) scar in the inferior wall (*arrowheads*), and subendocardial scar in the anterior wall (*arrow*)

30 Noncompaction Cardiomyopathy

Identify noncompaction morphology – heavily trabeculated endocardial layer, and a thinned, compacted epicardial layer.

Document segments involved.

Quantify ventricular volumes, systolic or diastolic dysfunction.

Look for associated abnormalities: ASD, VSD, aortic stenosis, and hypoplastic right heart syndromes.

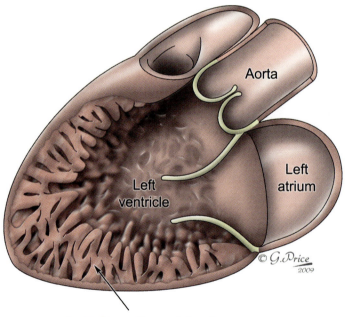

muscular wall consists of a
meshwork of numerous trabeculations

Fig. 30.1. Schematic illustration of non-compaction cardiomyopathy

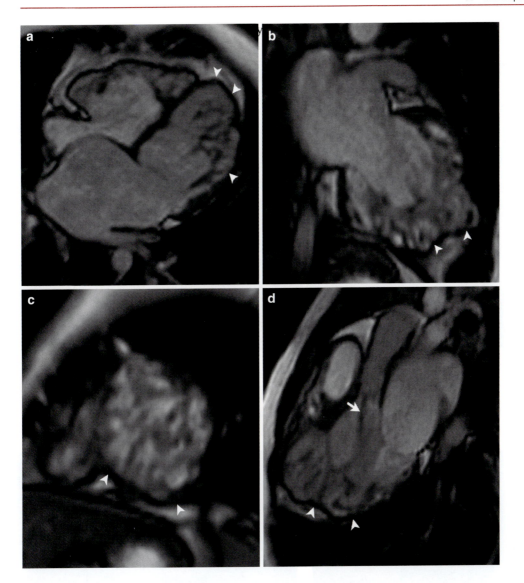

Fig. 30.2. b-SSFP images from a patient with LVNC (**a**) 4-Ch and (**b**) vertical long-axis views demonstrate severe left atrial dilatation, (**c**) short-axis, and (**d**) left ventricular-outflow compared to the thin layer of compacted myocardium (*arrowheads*). Incidental mild aortic valve regurgitation is also seen (*arrow*)

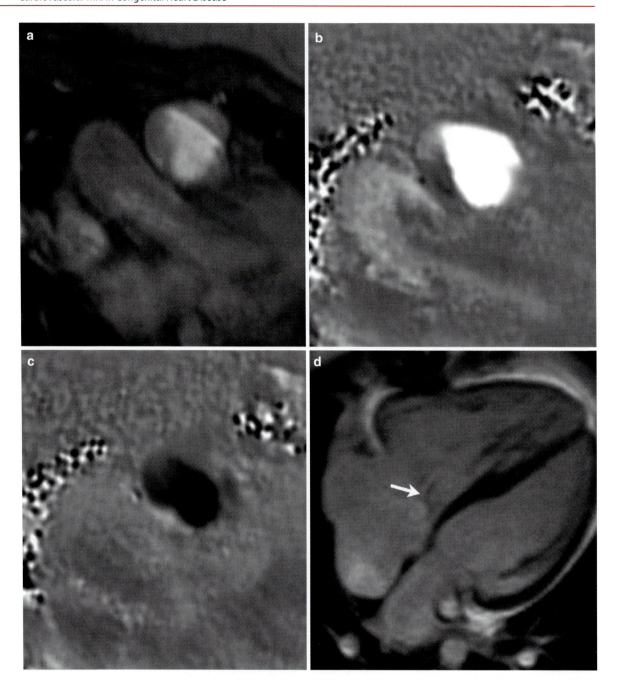

Fig. 32.4. Selected images in a patient with pulmonary regurgitation: (**a**) magnitude, (**b**) systolic, (**c**) diastolic phase contrast images, showing pulmonary regurgitation and (**d**) b-SSFP 4-Ch image showing a moderately dilated, and mildly hypertrophied right ventricle. Note the flattening of the interventricular septum, and dilated right atrium. A high signal jet of tricuspid regurgitation can also be seen (*arrow*)

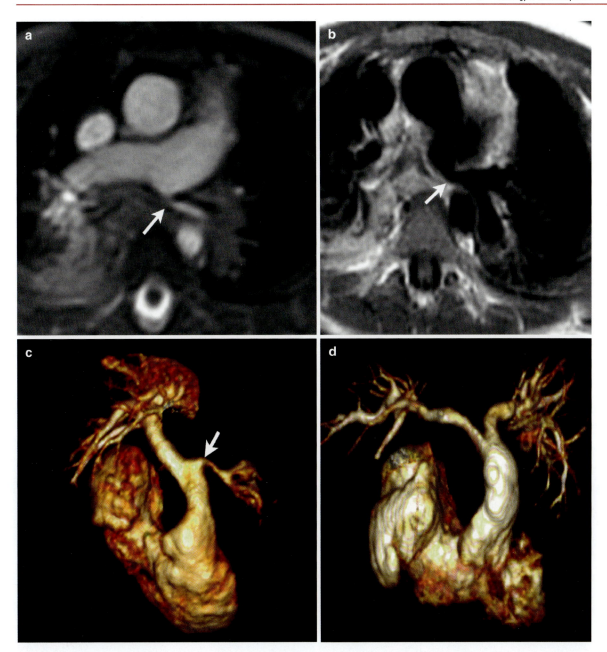

Fig. 32.5. Selected images showing branch pulmonary artery narrowing (**a**) b-SSFP axial image, (**b**) black-blood turbo spin echo, (**c**) volume-rendered 3D reconstruction of a contrast-enhanced MR angiogram showing LPA stenosis (*arrow*) and (**d**) volume-rendered 3D reconstruction of a CE-MRA showing bilateral narrowing of the pulmonary arteries. BT shunts had previously been present on both sides

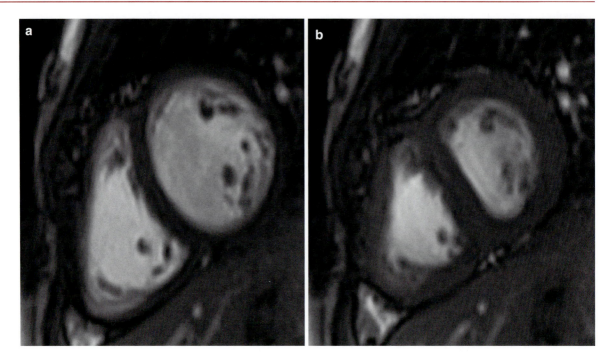

Fig. 32.6. b-SSFP images demonstrating systolic flattening of the interventricular septum in a patient with residual right ventricular outflow tract obstruction (**a**) diastolic, (**b**) systolic

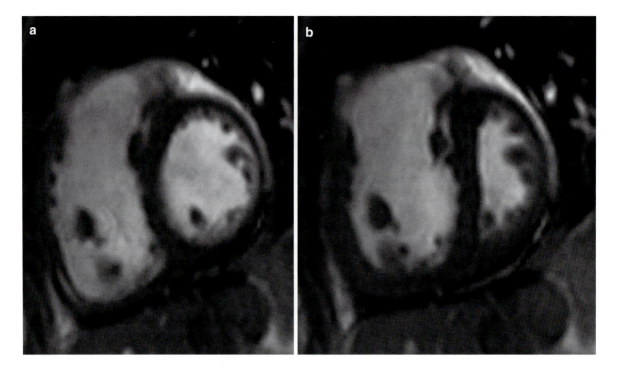

Fig. 32.7. Balanced-SSFP images demonstrating early diastolic flattening of the interventricular septum in a patient with severe pulmonary regurgitation (**a**) late diastolic (**b**) early diastolic

Notes

33   Pulmonary Stenosis

Visualise RVOT, MPA and branch PA morphology.

Describe mechanism of RVOTO – sub-valvar, valvar, supravalvar.

Measure valve annulus.

Assess post-stenotic dilatation of MPA.

Quantify valve stenosis and regurgitation.

Quantify RV volumes, systolic function, hypertrophy.

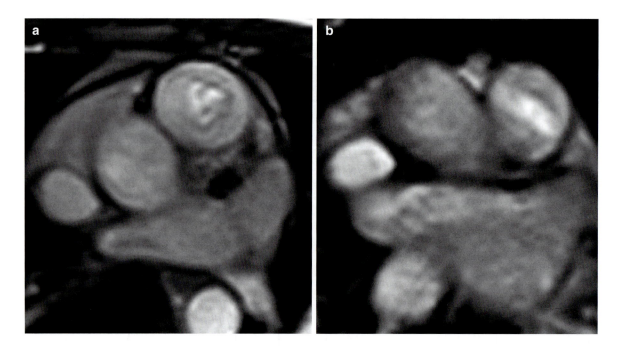

Fig. 33.1. b-SSFP en-face images of stenotic pulmonary valves (**a**) trileaflet valve (**b**) bicuspid valve

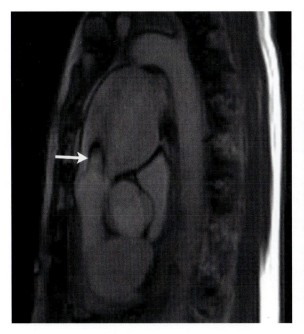

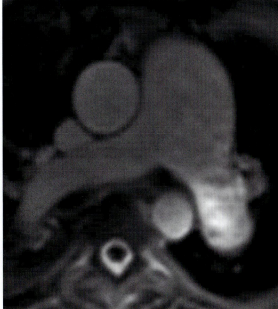

Fig. 33.2. b-SSFP image RVOT view, showing systolic flow acceleration (*arrow*) across the pulmonary valve into a severely dilated MPA

Fig. 33.3. b-SSFP axial image showing dilated MPA and branch pulmonary arteries

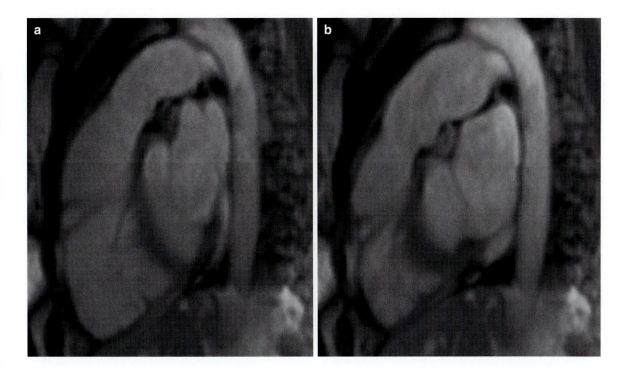

Fig. 33.4. b-SSFP images RVOT view of pulmonary stenosis following treatment with balloon valvuloplasty (**a**) diastole, (**b**) systole. Note the dynamic shape

34   Percutaneous Pulmonary Valve Implantation

Describe RVOT & pulmonary trunk morphology (size & shape) & dynamic nature.

Measure implantation site in systole and diastole – must be 14–22 mm in diameter.

Delineate coronary course and proximity to implantation site.

Post-implantation assess device stability & valve competence.

Quantify ventricular volumes and function.

Assess stent fractures using AP/lateral CXR.

Use CT for 3D visualisation of stent architecture.

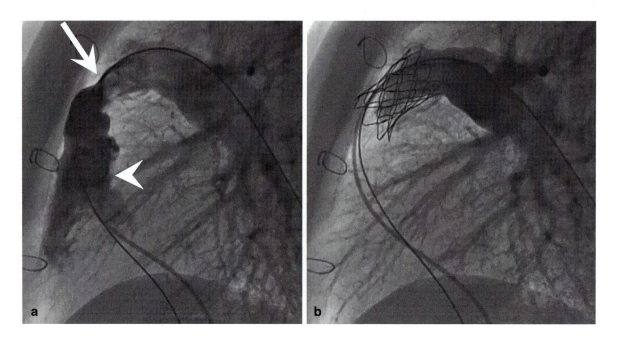

Fig. 34.1. Lateral catheter angiogram (**a**) pre-PPVI, showing stenosis (*arrow*) and PR (contrast in RV – *arrowhead*). (**b**) Post-PPVI, stenosis relieved, no PR

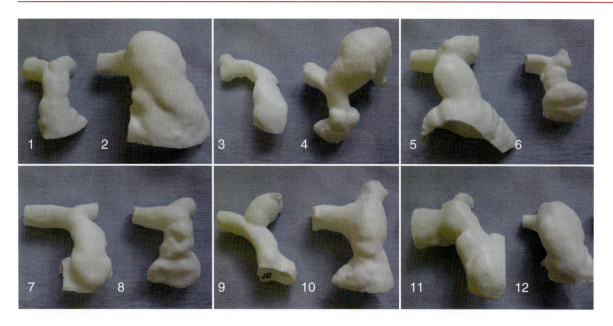

Fig. 34.2. 3D models reconstructed from CE-MRA. Twelve patients with ToF, treated with surgical correction as neonates. Note variation of RVOT anatomy, 12–15 years following neonatal surgery. Patients 1, 3, 4, 6 and 9 are suitable for PPVI

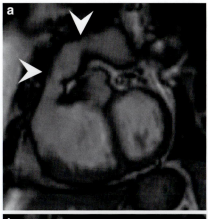

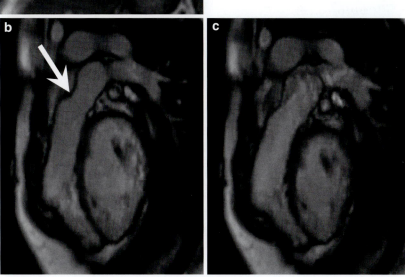

Fig. 34.3. b-SSFP frames from RVOT cine images. (**a**) Systolic frame (identical to diastolic frame) showing a fixed calcified conduit with two focal narrowing (*arrowheads*). (**b**, **c**) Diastolic and systolic frames from a different patient showing a potential narrowing (*arrow*) in diastole (**b**), which is dynamic and leaves no narrowing during systole (**c**)

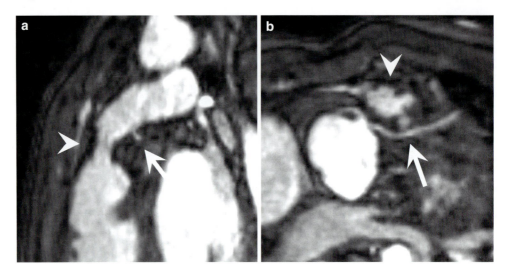

Fig. 34.4. Sagittal (**a**) and axial (**b**) reformats from a 3D b-SSFP whole-heart acquisition. In (**a**) the LCA (*arrow*) appears to be at some distance from the RVOT/pulmonary trunk narrowing (*arrowhead*); however in (**b**) the LCA (*arrow*) can be seen to be in very close proximity to the proposed site of PPVI. Test balloon expansion is required in this patient

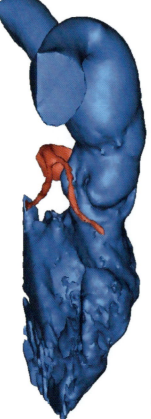

Fig. 34.5. Volume rendered 3D contrast enhanced CT showing the relationship of the LCA to the posterior surface of this dilated RVOT/pulmonary trunk

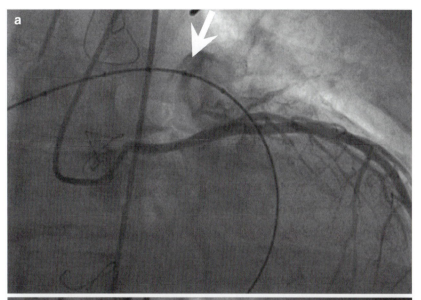

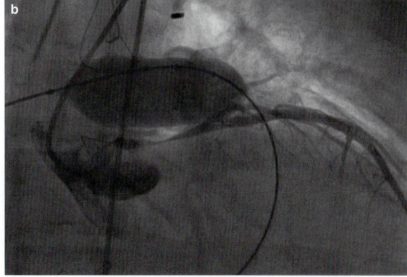

Fig. 34.6. Coronary artery angiogram before (**a**) and after ballon testing (b). In (a) circular homograft calcification can be clearly seen (*arrow*), and in (**b**) LCA compression. PPVI was not performed in this patient, who was referred for conventional surgical pulmonary valve replacement

35   Pulmonary Atresia and VSD

Characterise the presence or absence of native central PAs (supplied by a PDA or BT shunt).

Delineate number and course of multifocal pulmonary blood supply (MAPCAs).

Show relationship of MAPCAs to other structures: trachea, bronchi, oesophagus.

If dual blood supply is present, show relation of MAPCAs to "true" hypoplastic central PAs.

Quantify distance between neck of RVOT and PA confluence (this impacts surgical strategy or requirement for RV-PA conduit).

Post-op: assess RV-PA conduit function (valve regurgitation or stenosis).

Post-op: Quantify RV volumes, systolic function.

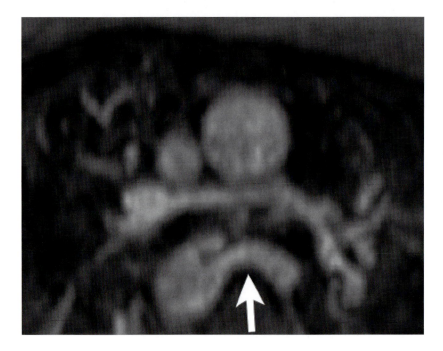

Fig. 35.1. Axial MIP from gadolinium enhanced MRA, showing that pulmonary arteries are disconnected from the RVOT, and that they are confluent and hypoplastic. Note the large MAPCA from the aorta to the left lung (*arrow*). All the pulmonary blood flow is via collateral vessels, some of which have anastomosed with the pulmonary arteries

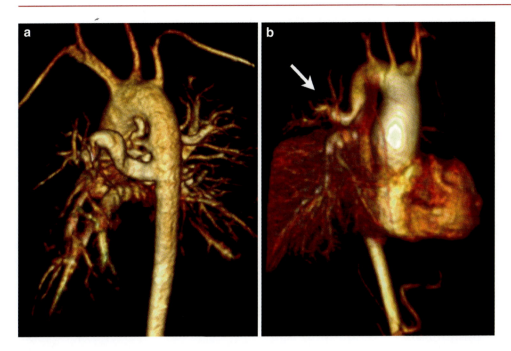

Fig. 35.2. Volume-rendered 3D reconstruction from gadolinium-enhanced MRA of the aorta showing large aortopulmonary collaterals (MAPCAs) supplying the lung (**a**). (**b**) The right upper lobe (*arrow*) is poorly perfused, demonstrating lobar pulmonary hypertension

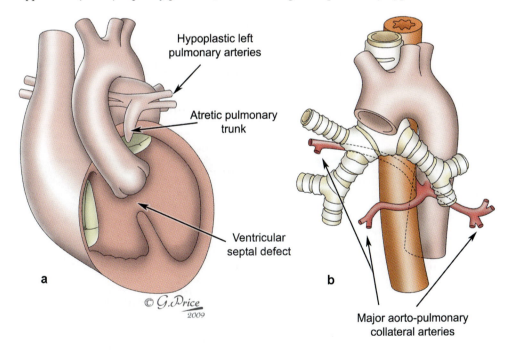

Fig. 35.3. (**a**)Schematic drawing of pulmonary atresia with VSD and MAPCA's. Note characteristic sub-aortic perimembranous VSD, the analogous anatomy to tetralogy of Fallot and the confluent pulmonary arteries. (**b**) Diagram showing relationship of great vessels to trachea (consider CT). Note the major aorto-pulmonary collateral arteries from the descending aorta providing pulmonary blood flow

36 Transposition of the Great Arteries: Arterial Switch Operation

Identify any RVOT obstruction, neo-pulmonary valve stenosis or supravalvar PS.

Identify any neo-aortic valve stenosis or supravalvar AS (surgical suture site).

Assess branch PAs – stenoses related to branch pulmonary artery distortion following the Le Compte procedure.

Quantify proportional flow in branch PAs.

Identify dilatation of ascending Ao (often at sites of coronary button transfer).

Assess ventricular function, volumes and RV mass (may be increased 2° RVOTO).

Assess coronary arteries – ostial stenosis, proximal kinking.

Identify regional wall-motion abnormalities or LGE evidence of previous infarction (following coronary distortion or compromise).

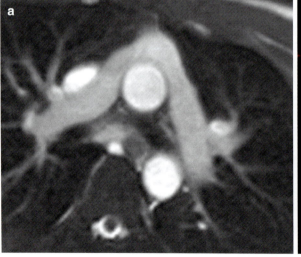
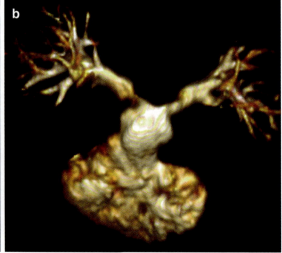

Fig. 36.1. b-SSFP images showing the pulmonary arteries straddling the aorta following the Le Compte procedure with (**a**) no narrowing of the pulmonary arteries, and (**b**) Volume-rendered 3D reconstruction of a contrast-enhanced MRA showing bilateral proximal branch pulmonary artery narrowing

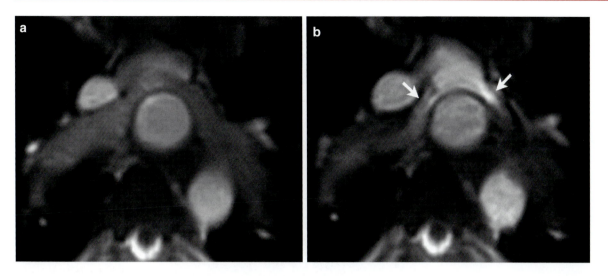

Fig. 36.2. b-SSFP images showing bilateral branch pulmonary artery narrowing (**a**) diastolic, and (**b**) systolic images. Note the flow acceleration (*arrows*)

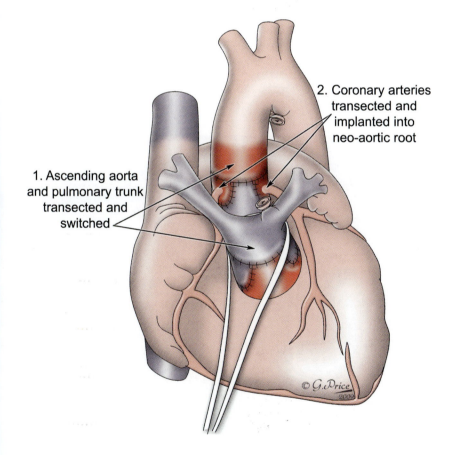

Fig. 36.3. Schematic drawing of Arterial Switch operation showing Le Compte manoeuvre with the translocation of aortic and pulmonary arteries. Note sites of coronary artery button removal and subsequent re-implantation into neo-aortic root

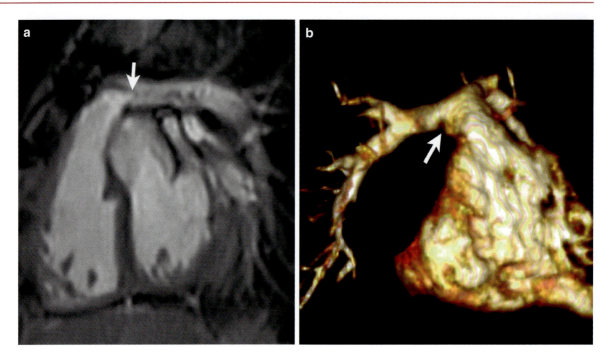

Fig. 36.4. Proximal kinking of the branch pulmonary arteries (**a**) b-SSFP image of the LPA with flow acceleration (*arrow*) (**b**) volume-rendered 3D reconstruction of a contrast-enhanced MR angiogram showing a proximal RPA kink (*arrow*)

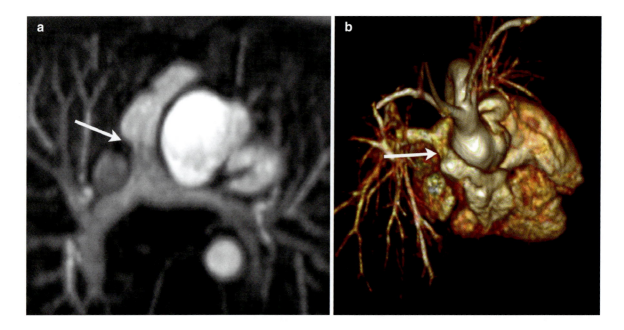

Fig. 36.5. Alternative arterial switch operation, with the main pulmonary artery (*arrow*) seen to pass on the right side, between the SVC, and aorta (**a**) axial MIP image from a contrast-enhanced MRA and (**b**) volume-rendered 3D reconstruction

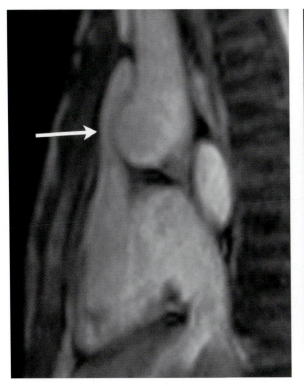

Fig. 36.6. b-SSFP image showing compression of the MPA (*arrow*) between the aorta and sternum

Fig. 36.7. Volume-rendered 3D reconstruction of a CE-MRA showing proximal LPA narrowing and narrowing of the ascending aorta at the site of anastomosis (*arrow*)

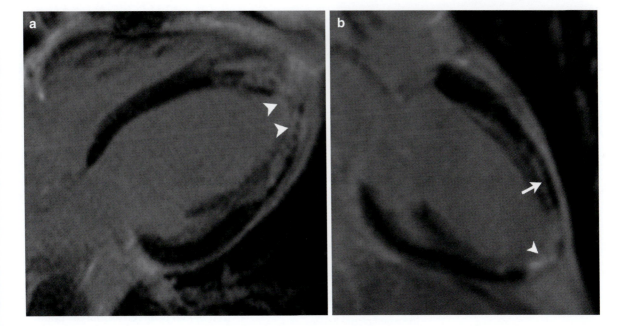

Fig. 36.8. CE-IR MRI images showing myocardial infarction (**a**) 4-Ch, (**b**) LV VLA. Note the full thickness enhancement in the apex (*arrowheads*), and subendocardial enhancement in the anterior wall (*arrow*)

37 Transposition of the Great Arteries: Senning and Mustard Repair

Assess patency of systemic venous pathways (degree of obstruction).

Assess patency of pulmonary venous pathway.

Quantify venous pathway obstruction with in-plane velocity. Look for loss of phasic flow or peak $V_{max} > 1.0$ m/s.

Assess integrity of atrial baffles or magnitude of baffle leak. There may be bidirectional shunting.

Look for azygous vein dilation 2° to baffle obstruction.

Assess ventricular function, volumes and RV mass (which will be increased 2° to systemic pressures).

Perform LGE to assess ventricular fibrosis/scar.

Note presence and severity of tricuspid valve regurgitation.

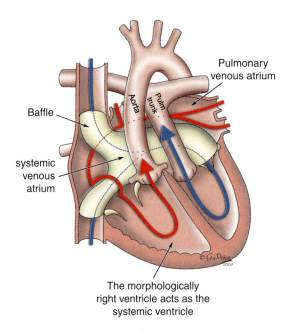

Pulmonary venous atrium

Baffle

systemic venous atrium

The morphologically right ventricle acts as the systemic ventricle

Fig. 37.1. Schematic drawing of an atrial switch (Mustard/Senning) for transposition of the great arteries. Note systemic (blue) blood is directed from the superior caval vein and inferior caval vein into the left atrium, then via the mitral valve to the left ventricle and then to the pulmonary artery. Pulmonary (red blood) is directed from the pulmonary veins to the right atrium, then via the tricuspid valve to the aorta

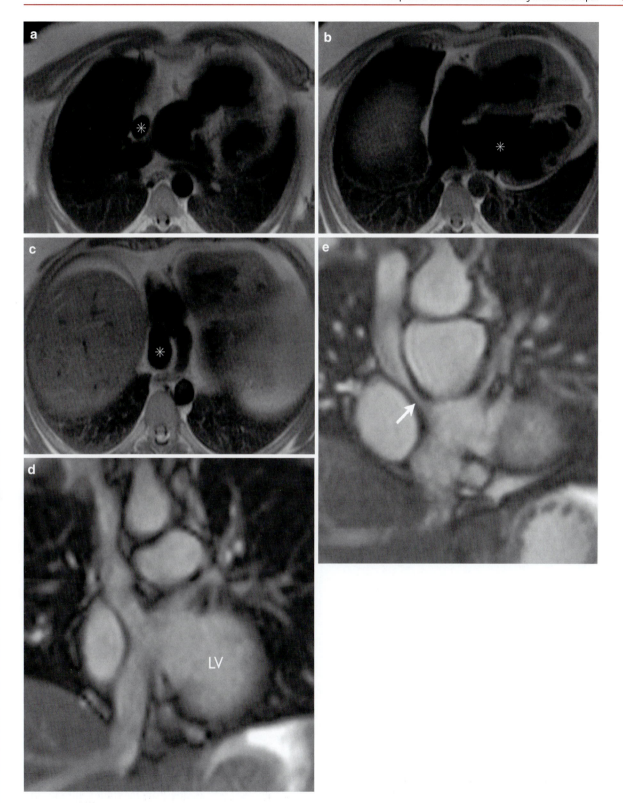

Fig. 37.2. While planning the image plane for the intra-atrial baffle, perform a three point plane (*asterisk*) in the following positions (**a**) SVC (**b**) mitral valve (**c**) IVC. This produces (**d**, **e**) b-SSFP image of systemic venous inflow to the left atrium: (**d**) unobstructed, (**e**) narrowed at the SVC to left atrium junction (*arrow*)

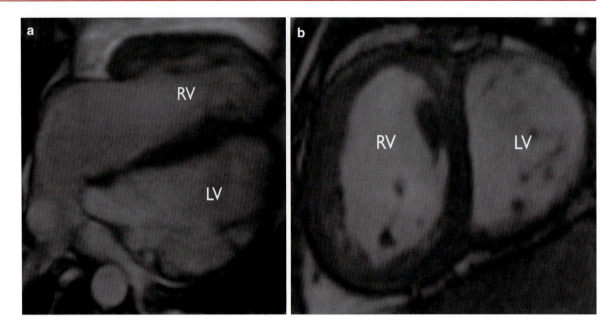

Fig. 37.3. b-SSFP images of a patient who has undergone the Mustard procedure (**a**) shows baffle taking pulmonary venous blood to the right atrium (**b**) short axis view shows expected hypertrophy of the systemic right ventricle. Note the bowing of the interventricular septum into the LV

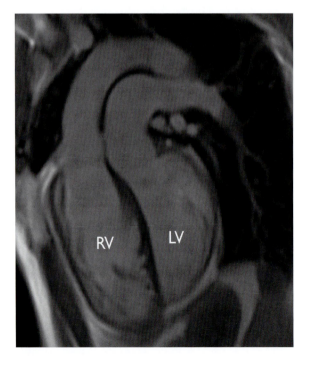

Fig. 37.4. b-SSFP images of a patient who has undergone the Mustard procedure. Oblique sagittal outlet view shows aorta arising from the right ventricle, and pulmonary artery arising posteriorly from the left ventricle

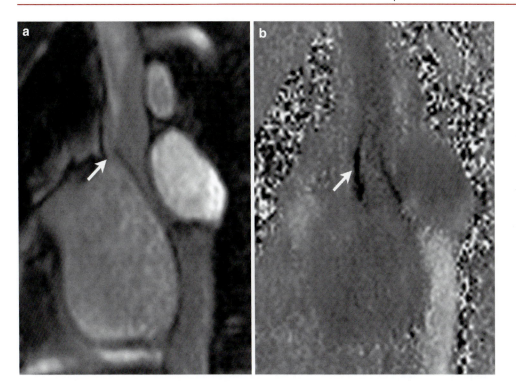

Fig. 37.5. Baffle leak (**a**) magnitude image shows discontinuity of the baffle at the junction of the SVC, and right atrium (*arrow*) (**b**) phase-contrast image shows flow (*arrow*) from the systemic veins into the right atrium (pulmonary venous chamber)

38 TGA with VSD and PS

Assess RV-PA conduit – stenosis and valve regurgitation can occur.

Look for conduit calcification, but it is better assessed by CT.

Assess branch pulmonary arteries – stenoses.

Look for LVOT obstruction – 2°VSD and/or VSD tunnel becoming restrictive.

Assess the integrity of VSD patch.

Assess ventricular function, volumes and mass – may be challenging due to the unusual position of the patch.

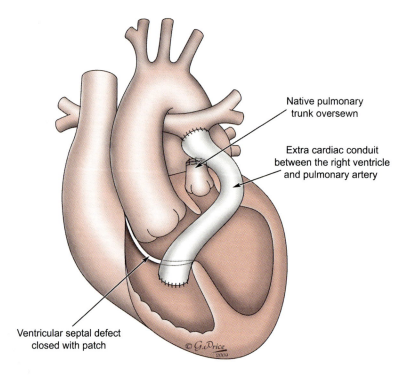

Native pulmonary trunk oversewn

Extra cardiac conduit between the right ventricle and pulmonary artery

Ventricular septal defect closed with patch

Fig. 38.1. Schematic drawing of Rastelli operation for transposition of the great arteries with ventricular septal defect and pulmonary stenosis

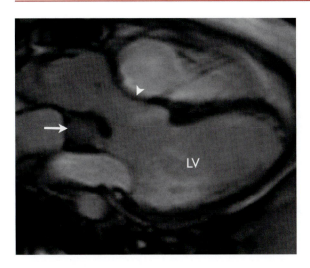

Fig. 38.2. b-SSFP image inflow/outflow view of the LV showing the VSD patch (*arrowhead*) in the RV used to create LVOT to the aorta. Note the oversewn hypoplastic pulmonary artery (*arrow*) between the aorta and LA

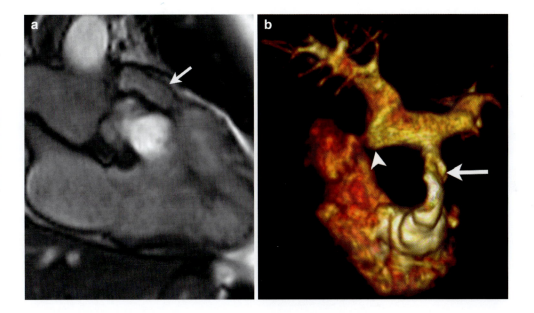

Fig. 38.3. Selected images showing RV-PA conduit narrowing. (**a**) b-SSFP image inflow/outflow view of the right ventricle showing a calcified (low signal) and narrowed RV-PA conduit (*arrow*) and (**b**) volume-rendered 3D reconstruction from gadolinium-enhanced MRA of the pulmonary arteries showing a narrowed and irregular RV-PA conduit inserting into the LPA. Note the native bifurcation to the right of this anastomosis

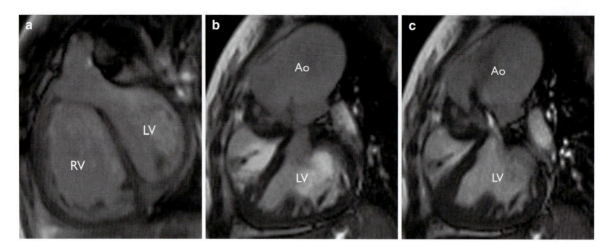

Fig. 38.4. b-SSFP short axis images of the VSD patch in an unobstructed outflow from the left ventricle to aorta (**a**), and in severe outflow obstruction caused by inward collapse of the VSD patch (**b**), diastolic and (**c**) systolic frames – note the post-stenotic dilatation of the ascending aorta

Notes

39 Congenitally Corrected Transposition of the Great Arteries

Describe A-V and V-A connections.

Look for VSD – present in 70% usually inlet associated with AV valve straddle.

Identify any outflow tract obstruction.

Describe tricuspid valve – possible Ebsteins malformation.

Perform late enhancement to assess for systemic RV fibrosis or scarring.

Look for associated anomalies – dextrocardia, RV inflow obstruction caused by supra-tricuspid ring), aortic arch hypoplasia (± CoA).

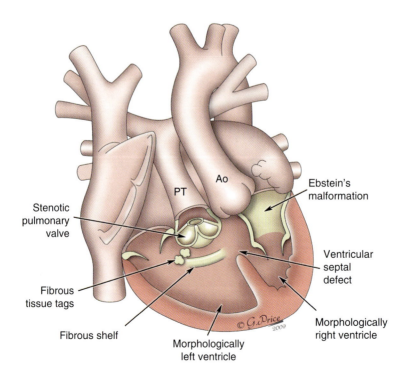

Fig. 39.1. Schematic drawing of congenitally corrected transposition

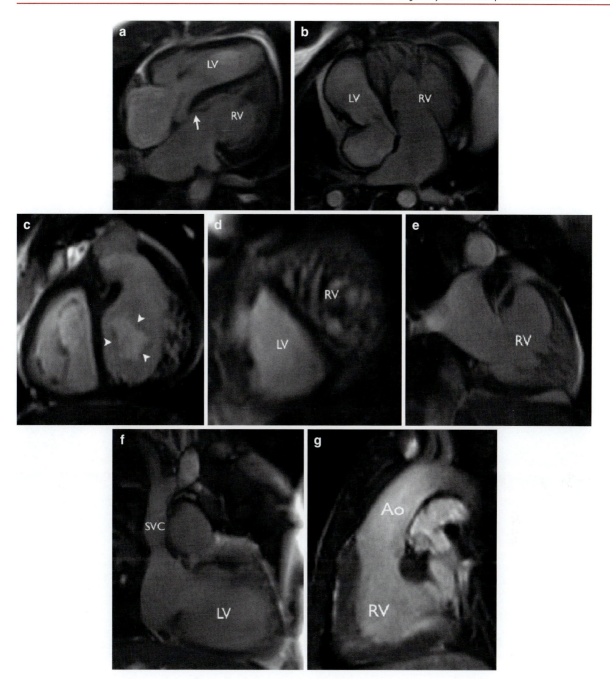

Fig. 39.2. (a) to (**g**) are b-SSFP images from several patients with CCTGA. (**a**) apical offset of the left-sided tricuspid valve (*arrow*), (**b**) 4-Ch showing moderate dilatation of the systemic RV, (**c**) SA view showing a left-sided tricuspid valve (*arrowheads*), and right-sided mitral valve, (**d**) SA view apical third, (**e**) VLA view showing pulmonary venous return to the RV, (**f**) VLA view showing systemic venous return to the left ventricle, (**g**) sagittal oblique view demonstrating systemic outflow from the RV

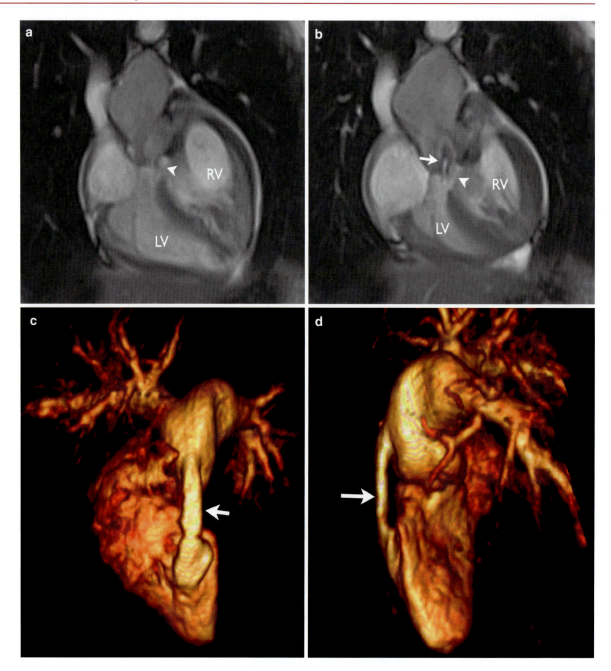

Fig. 39.3. Selected images from a patient with CCTGA with malaligned VSD (*arrowhead*), and pulmonary stenosis (**a**) diastolic and (**b**) systolic b-SSFP images, note the flow acceleration across the valve (*arrow*) in (**b**). Volume-rendered 3D reconstruction of a contrast-enhanced MRA anterior (**c**), and lateral (**d**) views showing an LV-PA conduit (*arrow*) to augment pulmonary blood flow and bypass the pulmonary stenosis

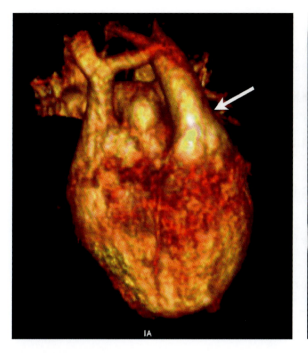

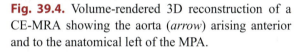

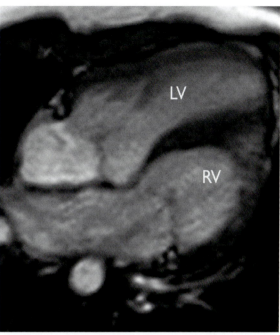

Fig. 39.4. Volume-rendered 3D reconstruction of a CE-MRA showing the aorta (*arrow*) arising anterior and to the anatomical left of the MPA.

Fig. 39.5. b-SSFP images in a patient with CCTGA and mild Ebstein's anomaly, with apical displacement of the septal leaflet of the tricuspid valve from the atrioventricular ring

40 Common Arterial Trunk

For non-repaired common arterial trunk delineate morphological sub-types:
- Type 1 PAs arise from main PA segment (usually left lateral aspect)
- Type 2 RPA & LPA arise from posterior wall of common trunk
- Type 3 RPA & LPA arise from lateral wall of common trunk

Evaluate functional status of truncal valve.

Describe size and position of VSD.

Look for associated anomalies – CoA, interruped aortic arch.

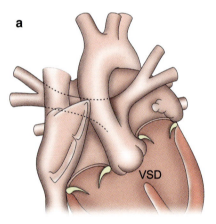

Type I - Pulmonary arteries arise
together from the posterior aspect
of the trunk and then divide

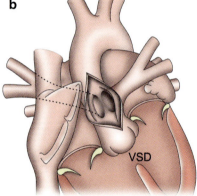

Type II - Pulmonary arteries arise
separately from the posterior
portion of the trunk

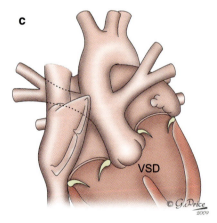

Type III - Pulmonary arteries arise
separately from the lateral
walls of the trunk

Fig. 40.1. Schematic drawing of common arterial trunk

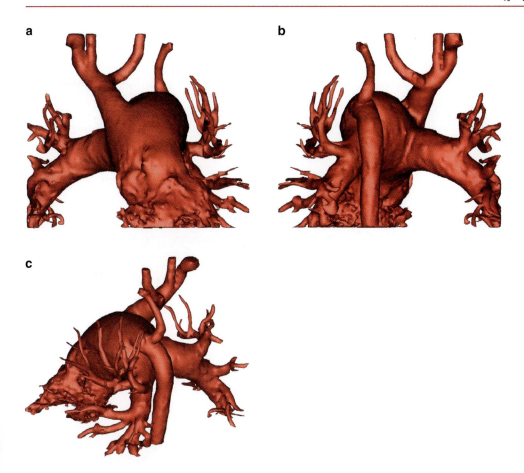

Fig. 40.2. Volume rendered contrast enhanced CT images of a patient with truncus arteriosus, confluence of the pulmonary arteries, and a Type B interruption of the aortic arch (**a**) anterior, (**b**) posterior and (**c**) posterior oblique views

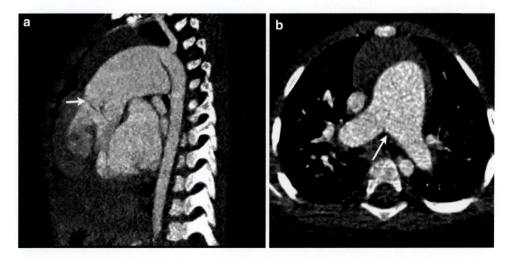

Fig. 40.3. (**a**) MPR axial image from a contrast enhanced CT in a patient with Type 2 truncus arteriosus and confluent pulmonary arteries (*arrow*). (**b**) MPR sagittal image from same patient. Note the common truncal valve overriding a VSD (*arrow*). The aorta continuity is maintained by a patent ductus arteriosus (*arrowhead*)

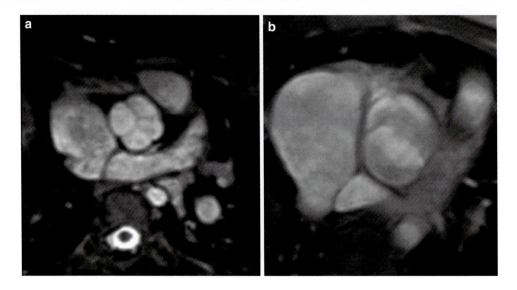

Fig. 40.4. b-SSFP images of the truncal valve (**a**) quadricuspid and (**b**) bicuspid – the truncal valve is most commonly tricuspid

Notes

41   Double Outlet Right Ventricle

Note great vessel arrangement – normal with sub-Ao VSD (Fallot type), anterior Ao with sub-pulmonary VSD (Taussig Bing type).

Describe VSD size, position and commitment.

Identify any associated outflow tract obstruction.

Assess ventricular function, volumes and mass (ventricles may be unbalanced).

Post-operatively evaluate for either a Fallot or TGA repair depending on initial DORV type.

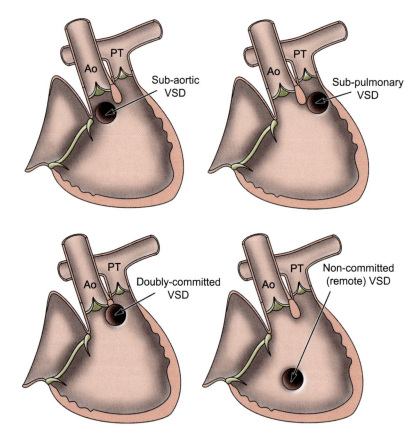

Fig. 41.1. Schematic diagrams of double outlet right ventricle with an anterior and rightward aorta. Note the variable position of the ventricular septal defect

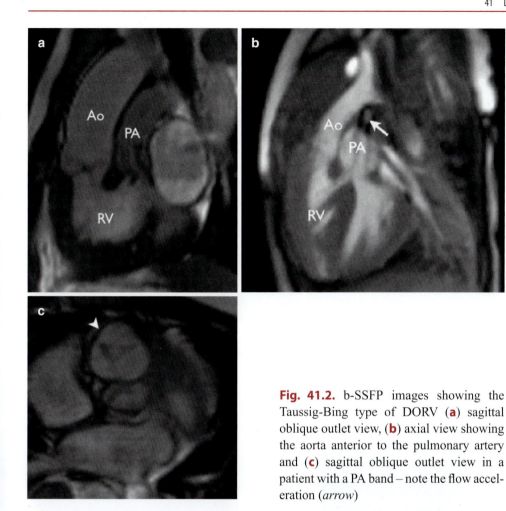

Fig. 41.2. b-SSFP images showing the Taussig-Bing type of DORV (**a**) sagittal oblique outlet view, (**b**) axial view showing the aorta anterior to the pulmonary artery and (**c**) sagittal oblique outlet view in a patient with a PA band – note the flow acceleration (*arrow*)

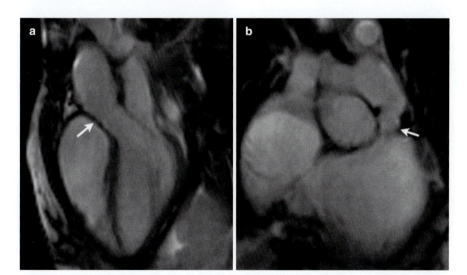

Fig. 41.3. b-SSFP images showing the Fallot type of DORV (**a**) LVOT view with a VSD patch (*arrow*), (**b**) RVOT view – note the sub-pulmonary narrowing (*arrow*)

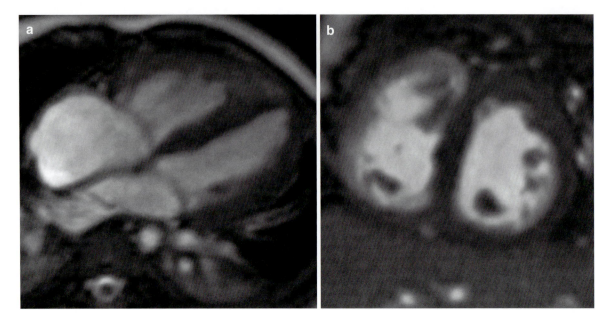

Fig. 41.4. b-SSFP images in a patient with unrepaired DORV. (**a**) 4-Ch view, (**b**) short axis view showing right ventricular hypertrophy

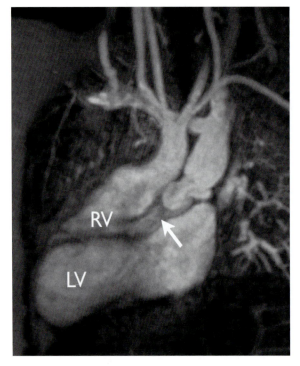

Fig. 41.5. 3D b-SSFP MIP image showing severe sub-pulmonary narrowing (*arrow*). The hypoplastic right ventricle is superior to the left ventricle

Notes

42 Double Inlet Left Ventricle

Describe AV valves – atrio-ventricular valve atresia or stenosis, with straddling of valve support apparatus across VSD.

Assess ventricular function and volumes – RV often rudimentary.

Evaluate septum – identify malalignment.

Determine AV valve competence.

Look for associated anomalies – double outlet great artery connection, PS, sub-Ao obstruction, & coarctation aorta can be present.

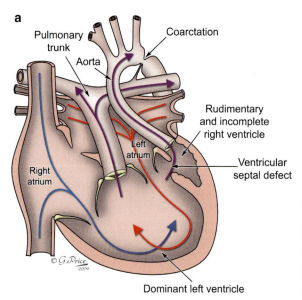
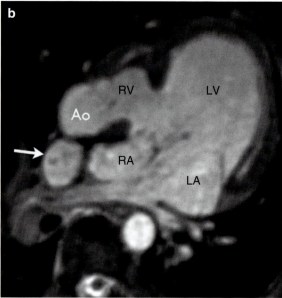

Fig. 42.1. (a) Schematic drawing showing double inlet left ventricle. Note the mixing of blue (systemic venous return) and red (pulmonary venous return) blood. Purple flow into the pulmonary artery from the left ventricle and aorta (via the ventricular septal defect and hypoplastic right ventricle). Also, note there is often an aortic coarctation. **(b)** 3D b-SSFP image showing DILV, and the aorta (Ao) arising from a hypoplastic RV. The patient has undergone a TCPC (arrow)

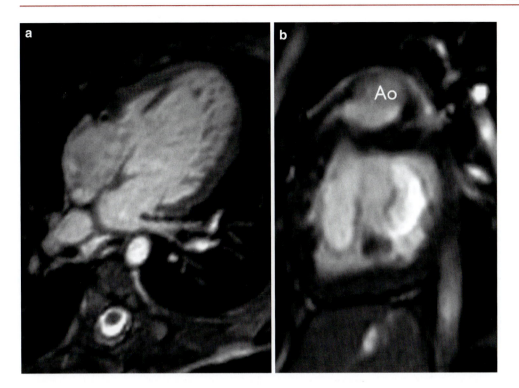

Fig. 42.2. b-SSFP images showing double inlet left ventricle, (**a**) oblique axial, (**b**) SA views –
the aorta can be seen arising superiorly from a rudimentary RV

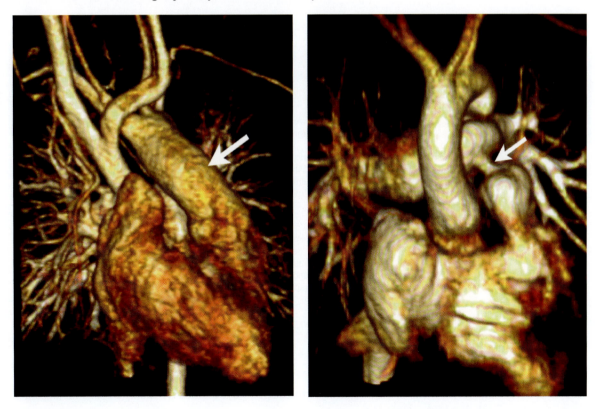

Fig. 42.3. Volume-rendered 3D reconstruction of a
CE-MRA showing transposed great vessels, with the
aorta arising from a hypoplastic RV (*arrow*)

Fig. 42.4. Volume-rendered 3D reconstruction of a
CE-MRA showing a pulmonary artery band (*arrow*)

43 Hypoplastic Left Heart Syndrome: Norwood Stage 1

Assess branch PA anatomy – including possible deformation at site of shunt insertion (modified BT or "Sano").

Assess arch reconstruction for residual obstruction or coarctation.

Assess right ventricular function and volume.

Identify any tricuspid valve regurgitation.

Identify any neo-aortic valve regurgitation.

Evaluate adequacy of atrial communication.

Look for veno-venous or aorto-pulmonary collateral vessels.

Look for bilateral SVCs.

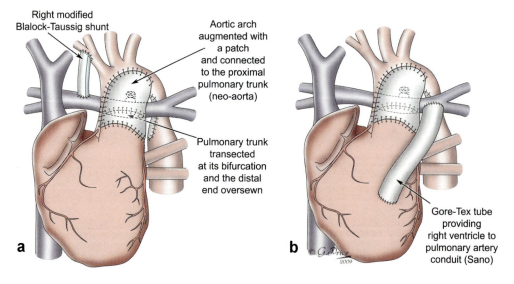

Fig. 43.1. Schematic drawing of Norwood stage 1. (**a**) Modified BT shunt, (**b**) Sano modification with RV to PA conduit

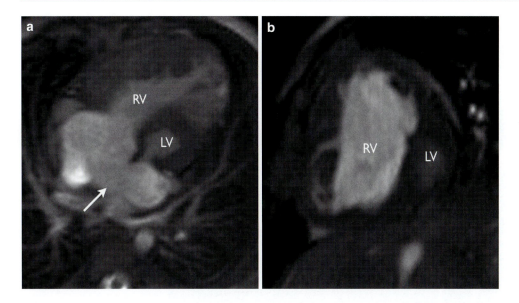

Fig. 43.2. b-SSFP images showing hypoplasia of the left ventricle, and servere hypertrophy of the systemic right ventricle (**a**) oblique axial- note the absence of atrial septum following atrial septectomy, (**b**) SA

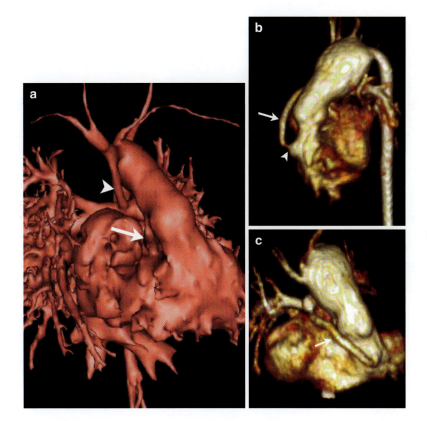

Fig. 43.3. Volume-rendered 3D reconstruction of CE-MRA (**a**) showing a DKS anastomosis connecting the native and neo-aorta (*arrow*) – anterior view, and modified BT shunt (*arrowhead*) (**b**) left and (**c**) right anterior oblique views – a deliberate kink has been left in the proximal Sano (*arrowhead*) to limit pulmonary blood flow

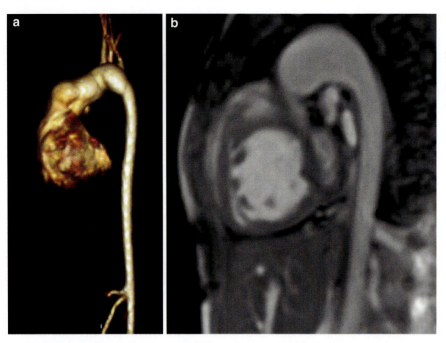

Fig. 43.4. Selected images showing a good aortic arch repair (**a**) volume-rendered 3D reconstruction of a CE-MRA and (**b**) sagittal oblique b-SSFP

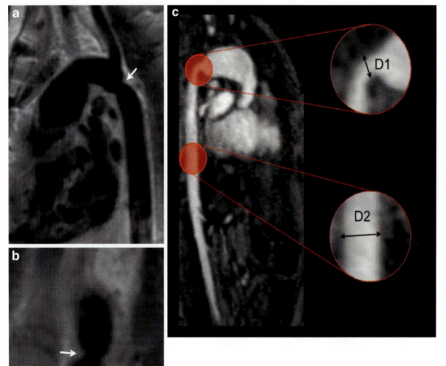

Fig. 43.5. Selected images showing moderate recoarctation (**a**) sagittal oblique, and (**b**) a cross-cut black blood turbo spin echo images, and (**c**) demonstrating one method of calculating the degree of recoarctation $(D2-D1)/D2 \times 100$

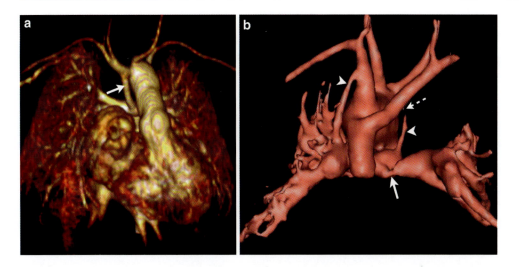

Fig. 43.6. Volume-rendered 3D reconstruction of a CE-MRA showing (**a**) unilateral and (**b**) bilateral BT shunts. In (**b**) note the severe proximal narrowing of the left BT shunt (*dashed arrow*), and narrowing of the proximal LPA (*arrow*)

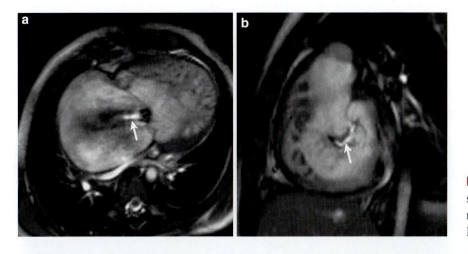

Fig. 43.7. b-SSFP image showing tricuspid valve regurgitation (*arrow*) (**a**) HLA, (**b**) SA views

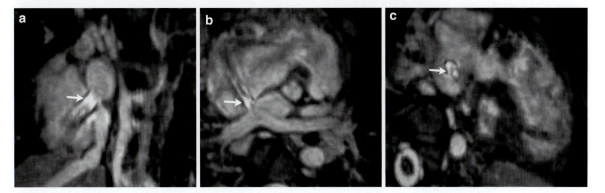

Fig. 43.8. Selected images showing a restrictive ASD with flow acceleration across the atrial septum (*arrow*), (**a–c**) 3D b-SSFP multiplanar cross-cuts

44   Bi-directional Cavo-pulmonary (Glenn) shunt

Assess branch PA anatomy and SVC-PA connection - look for stenosis.

Describe systemic venous return (SVC, IVC, hepatic veins).

Assess ventricular function and volume.

Identify any AV valve regurgitation.

Describe outflow tracts and arch.

Evaluate adequacy of atrial communication.

Look for veno-venous or aorto-pulmonary collateral vessels.

Assess pulmonary arterial pressure while the patient is under GA, by transducing the pressure in the internal jugular vein.

Identify any pulmonary vein stenosis.

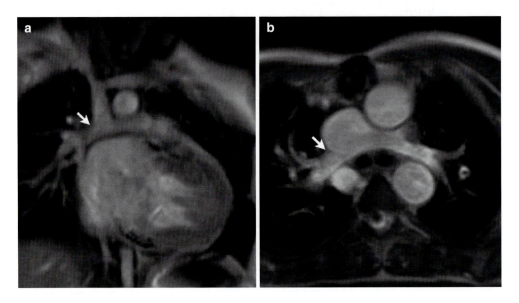

Fig. 44.1. b-SSFP image showing the BCPC anastomosis (*arrow*) between the superior vena cava and right pulmonary artery (**a**) coronal and (**b**) axial

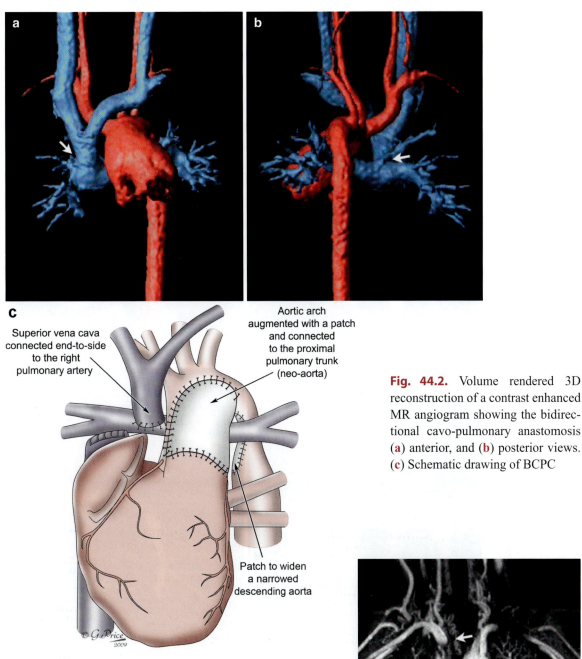

a

b

c

Superior vena cava
connected end-to-side
to the right
pulmonary artery

Aortic arch
augmented with a patch
and connected
to the proximal
pulmonary trunk
(neo-aorta)

Patch to widen
a narrowed
descending aorta

© G.Price
2009

Fig. 44.2. Volume rendered 3D reconstruction of a contrast enhanced MR angiogram showing the bidirectional cavo-pulmonary anastomosis (**a**) anterior, and (**b**) posterior views. (**c**) Schematic drawing of BCPC

Fig. 44.3. CE-MRA coronal MIP image showing multiple collaterals, (*arrows*) (systemic venous to pulmonary venous, and aortopulmonary), in a patient with a BCPC. Venous pressures precluded completion of the TCPC (Fontan) in this patient

45 Fontan-Type Circulation (Tricuspid Atresia)

Assess branch PA anatomy and RA-PA connection – look for stenosis.

Describe systemic venous return (SVC, IVC, hepatic veins).

Assess ventricular function and volume.

Identify any AV valve regurgitation.

Look for thrombus in RA.

Evaluate adequacy of atrial communication.

Look for veno-venous or aorto-pulmonary collateral vessels.

Assess pulmonary arterial pressure while the patient is under GA, by transducing the pressure in the internal jugular vein.

Identify any pulmonary vein stenosis.

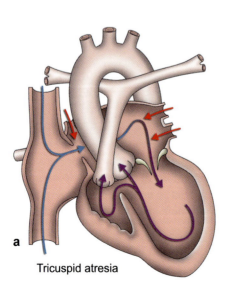

Tricuspid atresia

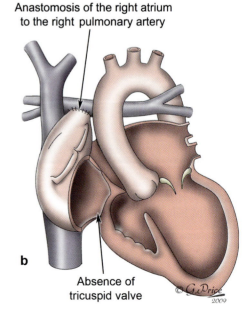

Anastomosis of the right atrium to the right pulmonary artery

Absence of tricuspid valve

Fig. 45.1. Schematic drawing of tricuspid atresia, (**a**) native anatomy and (**b**) following classical atrial pulmonary connection (APC) 'classical' Fontan

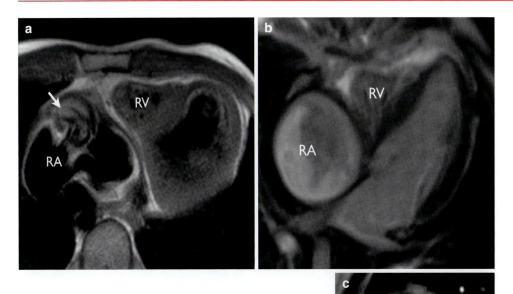

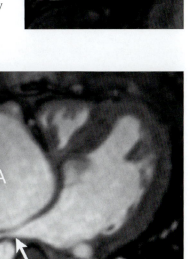

Fig. 45.2. Selected images in a patient with tricuspid atresia (**a**) black blood turbo spin echo showing high signal in the right atrium (*arrow*) caused by in plane swirling of blood, but must exclude thrombus. Also note the fat in the atrioventricular groove (*arrow*) separating the RA from RV. (**b**) b-SSFP image, at the same level as (a), showing a dilated RA, and hypoplastic RV. (**c**) SA view showing absence of the tricuspid valve

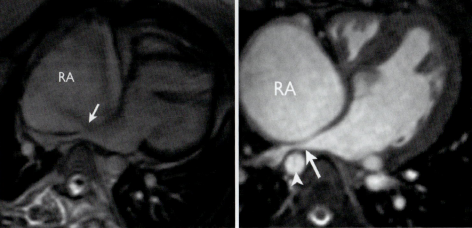

Fig. 45.3. (**a**) b-SSFP image showing an atrial septal defect with flow across the atrial septum. (**b**) 3D b-SSFP image showing a dilated RA with compression of the right lower lobe pulmonary veins (*arrow*), between the RA and right-sided descending thoracic aorta (*arrowhead*)

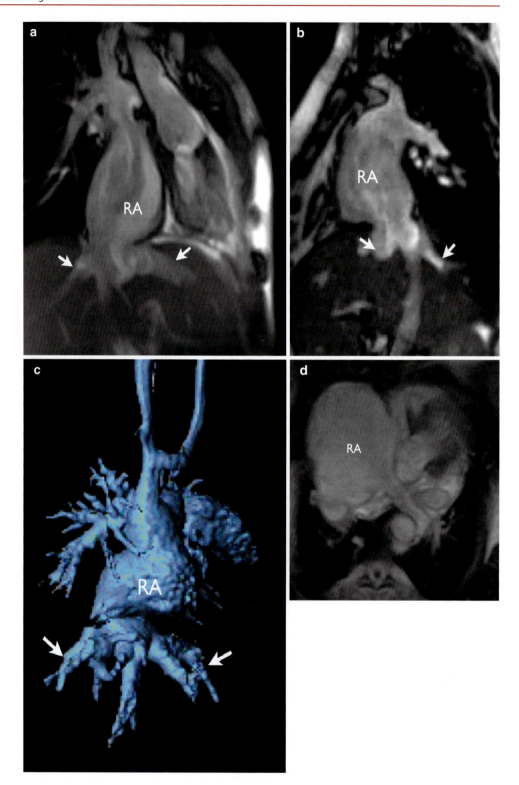

Fig. 45.4. b-SSFP image showing the atrio-pulmonary Fontan in three different patients. (**a**) Coronal, (**b**) sagittal and (**c**) axial views. Note the severe dilatation of the right atrium, and hepatic veins (*arrowheads*). (**d**) Volume rendered 3D reconstruction of a contrast enhanced MR angiogram showing the atriopulmonary Fontan. Note the severe dilatation of the RA, and hepatic veins (*arrows*)

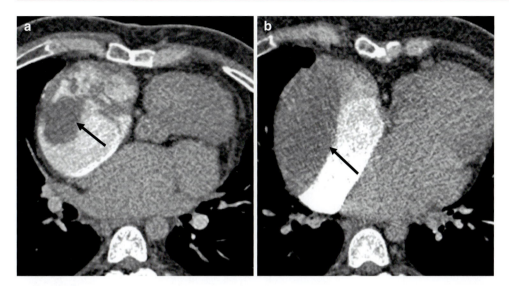

Fig. 45.5. (a) and (**b**) CE enhanced axial CT images, demonstrating large clot (*arrows*) in the right atrium

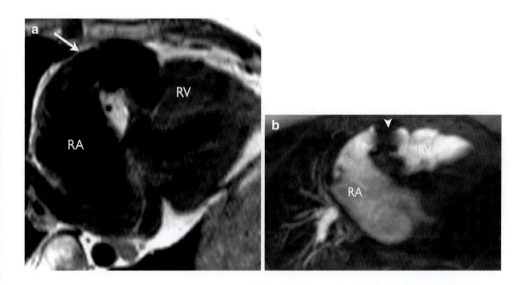

Fig. 45.6. HLA images of the Bjork modification of the Fontan with a conduit connection between the right atrium and hypoplastic right ventricle (**a**) black blood turbo spin echo and (**b**) CE-MRA axial MIP image at the same level as (**a**) showing a valved stent in situ (*arrow*)

46 Total Cavo-pulmonary Connection

Assess branch PA anatomy – look for stenosis.

Assess SVC-PA and IVC-PA connection – exclude stenosis, presence of thrombus.

Assess ventricular function and volume.

Identify any AV valve regurgitation.

Evaluate flow in fenestration between conduit and RA if present.

Evaluate adequacy of atrial communication.

Look for veno-venous or aorto-pulmonary collateral vessels.

Assess pulmonary arterial pressure while the patient is under GA, by transducing the pressure in the internal jugular vein.

Identify any pleural effusions and ascites indicating the presence of protein losing enteropathy (PLE), a sign of poor prognosis.

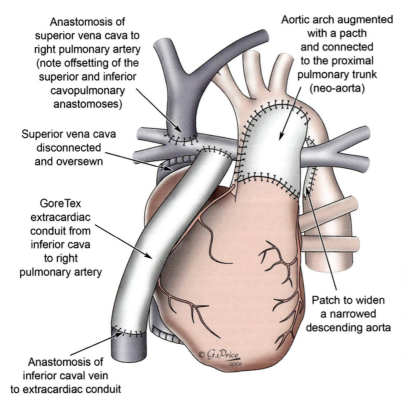

Anastomosis of superior vena cava to right pulmonary artery (note offsetting of the superior and inferior cavopulmonary anastomoses)

Superior vena cava disconnected and oversewn

GoreTex extracardiac conduit from inferior cava to right pulmonary artery

Anastomosis of inferior caval vein to extracardiac conduit

Aortic arch augmented with a pacth and connected to the proximal pulmonary trunk (neo-aorta)

Patch to widen a narrowed descending aorta

© G. Price 2009

Fig. 46.1. Schematic drawing of Total Cavo-pulmonary Connection in a patient with hypoplastic left heart syndrome. Note off-setting between Glenn and IVC-PA connection limiting flow related energy loss of directly opposing streams

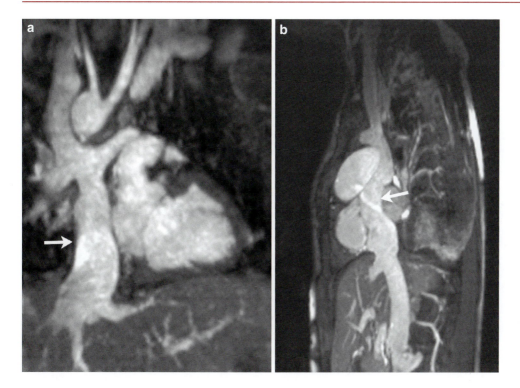

Fig. 46.2. 3D b-SSFP images showing a lateral tunnel TCPC (*arrow*). (**a**) Coronal MIP – note the offset of the IVC and SVC connections to the pulmonary artery, (**b**) sagittal MIP

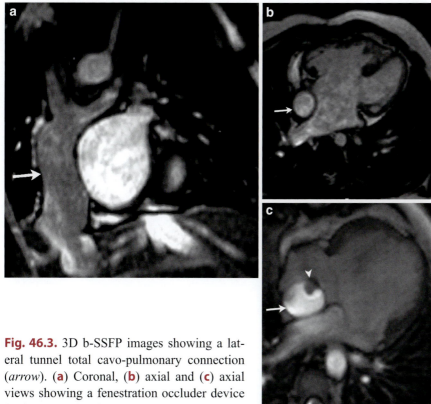

Fig. 46.3. 3D b-SSFP images showing a lateral tunnel total cavo-pulmonary connection (*arrow*). (**a**) Coronal, (**b**) axial and (**c**) axial views showing a fenestration occluder device in situ (*arrowhead*)

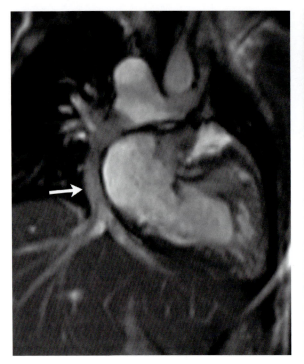

Fig. 46.4. b-SSFP image showing an extra cardiac conduit TCPC (*arrow*)

Fig. 46.5. Volume rendered 3D reconstruction of a CE-MRA showing a lateral tunnel total cavopulmonary connection (*arrow*) to the right pulmonary artery (*arrowhead*)

Fig. 46.6. b-SSFP image showing severe ascites (*arrow*), and a right pleural effusion (*arrowhead*) in a patient with a failing Fontan circulation and protein losing enteropathy

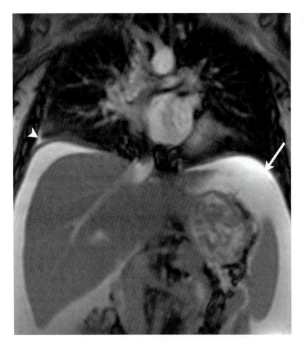

Notes

47   Anomalous Coronary Arteries

Delineate coronary artery anatomy – CT may be better.

Look for myocardial perfusion defects.

Identify areas of regional wall motion defects.

Assess ventricular function, volumes and LV mass.

Perform LGE – to determine infarct size if present.

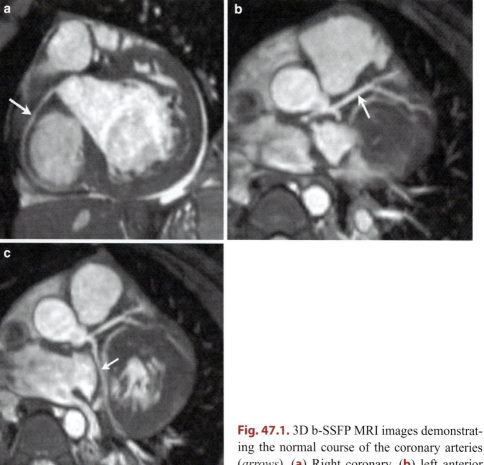

Fig. 47.1. 3D b-SSFP MRI images demonstrating the normal course of the coronary arteries (*arrows*). (**a**) Right coronary, (**b**) left anterior descending and (**c**) lateral circumflex

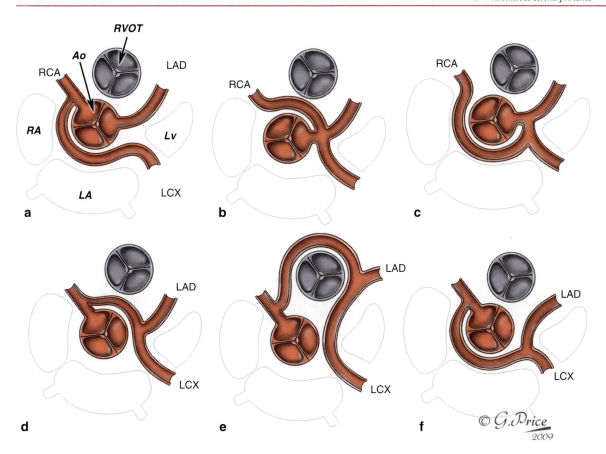

Fig. 47.2. Anatomic representation of the coronary arteries viewed in the oblique axial plane on MRI. RA=right atrium, LA=left atriuim, LV=left ventricle, Ao=aorta, RVOT=right ventricular outflow tract, LAD=left anterior descending artery, RCA=right coronary artery, LCX=left circumflex artery. (**a**) anomalous LCX from RCA (**b**) anomalous RCA from left main stem (LMS) with interarterial course between pulmonary trunk and aorta (**c**) anomalous RCA from LMS passing posteriorly between aorta and atria (**d**) anomalous left coronary artery arising from RCA with interarterial course between pulmonary trunk and aorta (**e**) anomalous left coronary artery arising from RCA passing posteriorly between aorta and atria (**f**) anomalous left coronary artery arising from RCA passing anterior to pulmonary trunk

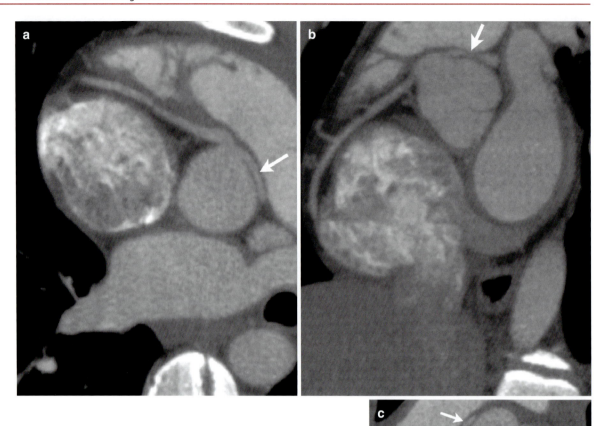

Fig. 47.3. MIP images from a cardiac gated contrast enhanced CT demonstrating anomalous origin of the left main stem (*arrow*) from the right coronary cusp, with a "malignant" course passing between the aorta and main pulmonary artery. (**a**) axial, (**b**) coronal oblique, (**c**) sagittal oblique

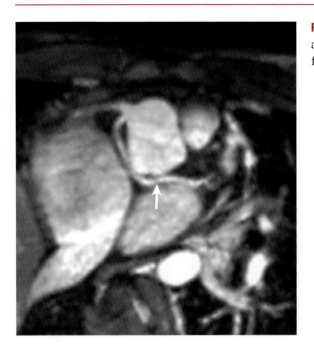

Fig. 47.4. 3D b-SSFP MIP image demonstrating anomalous origin of the lateral circumflex (*arrow*) from the right coronary cusp

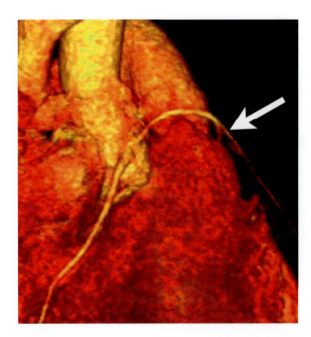

Fig. 47.5. Volume rendered cardiac gated CE-CT demonstrating anomalous origin of the left main stem from the right coronary cusp, with a "benign" course passing anterior to the main pulmonary artery. However, this course needs to be identified prior to any surgery of the RVOT, which can potentially be transected causing septal/ anterior LV infarction

48 Anomalous Left Coronary Artery from Pulmonary Artery

Describe coronary artery anatomy and origin of LCA from pulmonary artery.

Assess ventricular function and volumes – dilation and poor function due to ischaemia.

Identify mitral regurgitation – secondary to ischaemia.

Look for regional wall motion abnormalities.

Look for retrograde or bidirectional flow seen in proximal LCA (best seen with echocardiography).

Post-repair, look for supravalvar PS at site of PA patch repair, LV volumes and systolic function. Quantify mitral valve regurgitation.

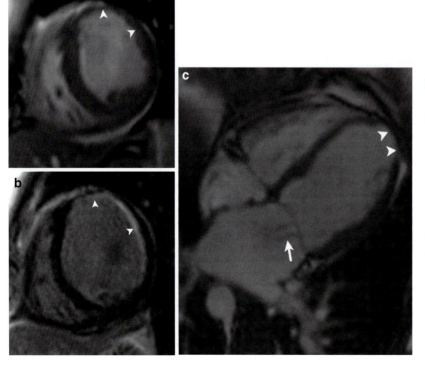

Fig. 48.1. SA views demonstrating myocardial infarction. (**a**) Systolic frame b-SSFP image shows thinning and akinesia of the anterior and lateral walls, (**b**) LGE MR image at the same level shows full thickness scar in the anterior wall, with a thick region of sub-endocardial scar extending down the lateral wall. (**c**) b-SSFP image 4-Ch view demonstrates ischeamic dilatation of the left ventricle, with thinning of the apex (*arrowheads*), and mitral regurgitation (*arrows*)

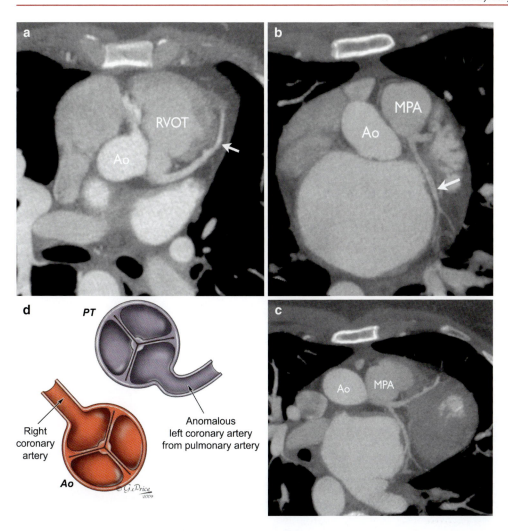

Fig. 48.2. Contrast enhanced cardiac gated CT MIP images, showing anomalous origin of the left coronary artery from the pulmonary artery (**a**) left anterior descending artery (LAD), (**b**) lateral circumflex artery, and (**c**) left main stem bifurcating into LAD and lateral circumflex arteries. Note the right coronary artery arises normally. (**d**) Schematic drawing of ALCAPA

49 Kawasaki Disease

Delineate coronary course and aneurysms – coronary stenoses are best seen on catheter coronary angiography or coronary CT.

Document aneurysms – number, site, size.

Identify thrombus formation within aneurysm.

Assess ventricular function, volumes and regional wall motion abnormalities.

Perform LGE – segmental endocardial fibrosis or scarring.

Identify myocardial perfusion defects.

Quantify associated mitral regurgitation or aortic regurgitation.

Visualize other possibly affected vessels – axillary, femoral, carotid, renal arteries.

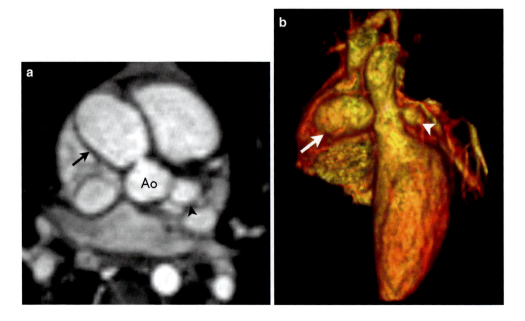

Fig. 49.1. Massive coronary artery aneurysms of RCA (*arrow*) and LMS (*arrowhead*) in an 8-year old boy with Kawasaki disease. (**a**) 3D b-SSFP image, (**b**) volume rendered image

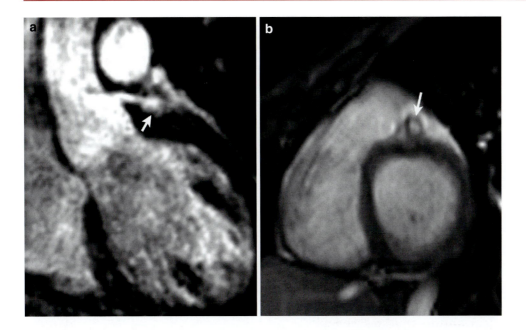

Fig. 49.2. Aneurysm of the LAD artery (*arrow*). (**a**) 3D b-SSFP image, (**b**) SA cine

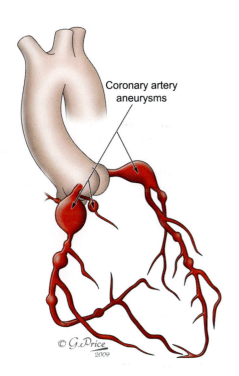

Fig. 49.3. Schematic drawing of Kawasaki disease

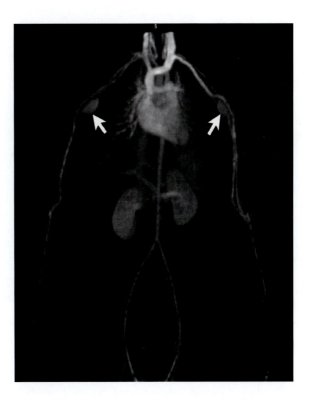

Fig. 49.4. 3D MIP reconstruction of a CE-MR angiogram in a patient with bilateral axillary artery aneurysms (*arrows*)

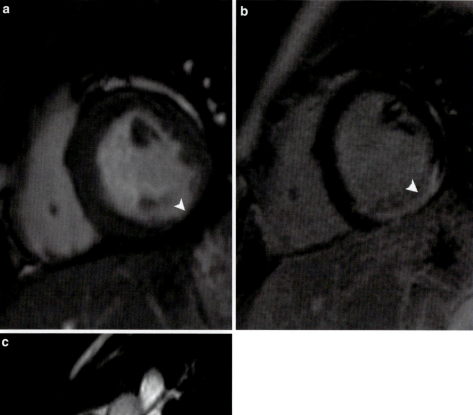

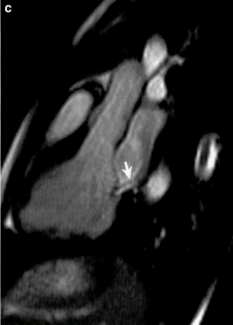

Fig. 49.5. SA views demonstrating myocardial infarction. (**a**) Systolic frame b-SSFP image shows thinning and akinesia of the inferior wall (*arrowheads*). (**b**) CE-IR MRI image at the same level shows full thickness scar in the inferior wall (*arrowhead*), (**c**) balanced-SSFP image of left ventricular outflow tract view shows mild mitral regurgitation due to papillary muscle ischaemia (*arrow*)

Notes

50 Total Anomalous Pulmonary Venous Drainage

Describe pulmonary venous drainage:
- Supracardiac drainage: vertical vein to right SVC, innominate vein
- Intracardiac drainage: to coronary sinus, or directly to RA
- Infracardiac drainage: towards diaphragm into portal or hepatic venous system
- *Mixed Type:* drainage of left & right sided veins to differing sites

Identify areas of pulmonary venous obstruction.

Confirm obligatory R to L shunt at atrial level.

Look for associated anomalies – right atrial isomerism.

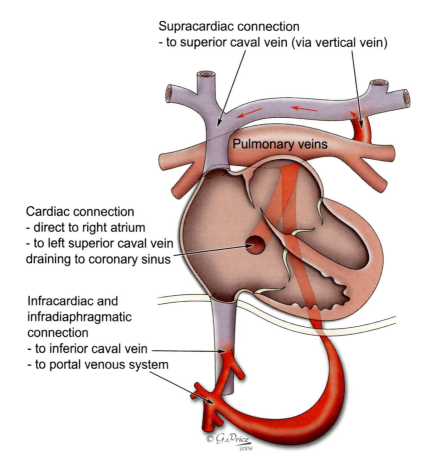

Supracardiac connection
- to superior caval vein (via vertical vein)

Pulmonary veins

Cardiac connection
- direct to right atrium
- to left superior caval vein
draining to coronary sinus

Infracardiac and
infradiaphragmatic
connection
- to inferior caval vein
- to portal venous system

© G.Price
2009

Fig. 50.1. Schematic drawing of total anomalous pulmonary venous drainage

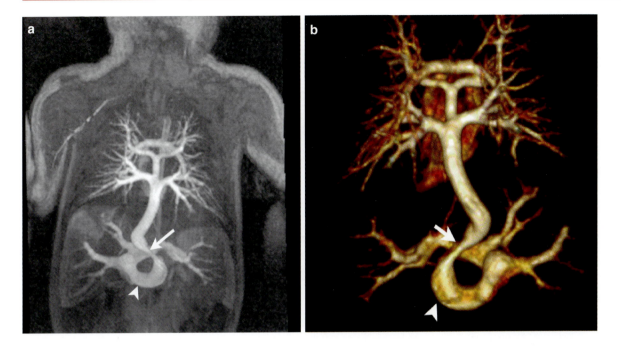

Fig. 50.2. CE-MRA showing total anomalous infracardiac drainage of the pulmonary veins – note the narrowing of the veins as they pass through the diaphragm (*arrow*) before draining into the portal vein (*arrowhead*). (**a**) Coronal MIP, (**b**) volume rendered 3D reconstruction

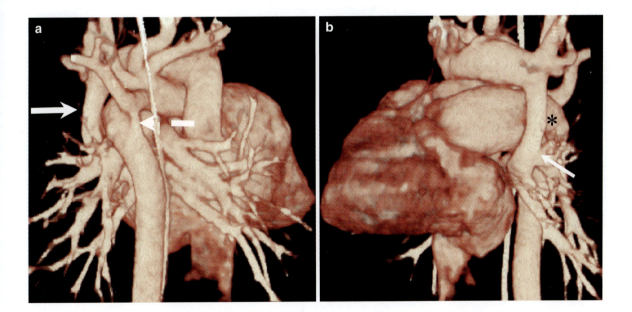

Fig. 50.3. CE-MRA showing total anomalous supracardiac drainage of the pulmonary veins (*arrow*) – note also the aortic coarctation (*dashed arrow*), and the large patent ductus arteriosus (*asterisk*). (**a**) Posterior and (**b**) left lateral volume rendered 3D reconstruction

51 Partial Anomalous Pulmonary Venous Drainage

Describe pulmonary venous drainage:
- Right upper lobe veins drain into SVC. This type is associated with sinus venosus ASD.
- Left upper lobe veins often drain into innominate vein.
- Right lower lobe veins can drain into IVC (scimitar vein) or to hepatic or portal veins.

Assess branch PAs – can be associated with hypoplastic branch PAs and lung.

Quantify ventricular volumes and function and assess RA dilation.

Quantify Qp:Qs.

Suspect if high Qp:Qs and no ASD or VSD.

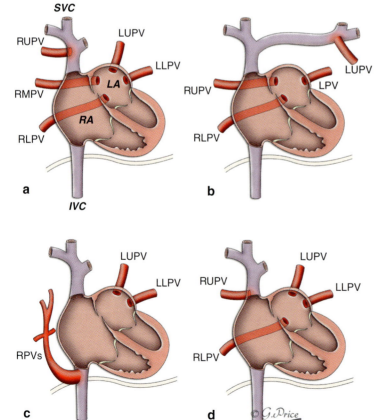

Fig. 51.1. Schematic drawing of partially anomalous pulmonary venous drainage. SVC=superior caval vein, IVC=inferior caval vein, RA=right atrium, LA=left atrium, RUPV=right upper pulmonary vein, RMPV=right middle pulmonary vein, RLPV=right lower pulmonary vein, LUPV=left upper pulmonary vein, LLPV=left lower pulmonary vein (**a**) RUPV to SVC, note presence of three right sided pulmonary veins (**b**) LUPV to brachiocephalic vein, (**c**) scimitar vein to IVC, (**d**) RUPV to SVC

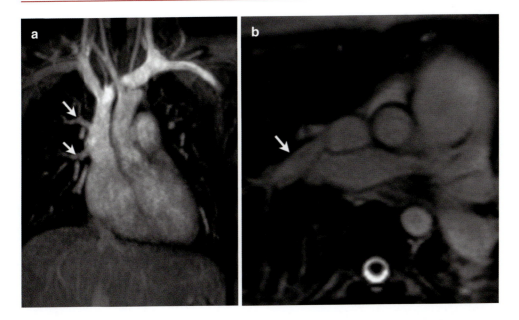

Fig. 51.2. (a) CE-MR angiogram coronal MIP image showing partial anomalous drainage of the right upper and middle pulmonary veins (*arrows*) into the superior vena cava. (**b**) b-SSFP image showing anomalous drainage of the right upper pulmonary vein (*arrows*) into the superior vena cava

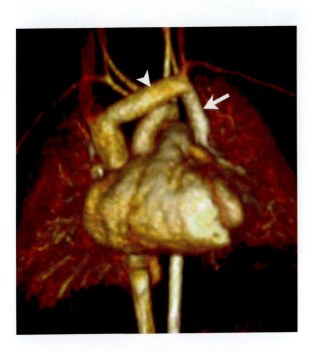

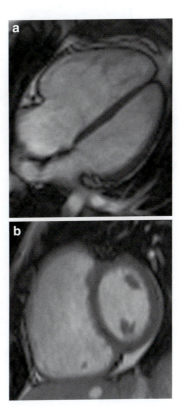

Fig. 51.3. Volume rendered 3D reconstruction of a CE-MRA showing partial anomalous drainage of the left upper lobe pulmonary veins (*arrow*) into the innominate vein (*arrowhead*)

Fig. 51.4. b-SSFP image showing a dilated right ventricle. (**a**) 4-Ch and (**b**) SA in a patient with a Qp:Qs of 3:1

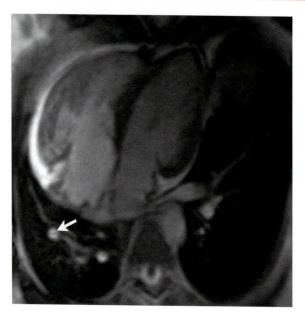

Fig. 51.5. b-SSFP 4-Ch image in a patient with Scimitar syndrome – note the dilated right ventricle, the enlarged right lower lobe pulmonary vein (*arrow*), and hypoplasia of the right lung with the heart shifted to the right hemithorax

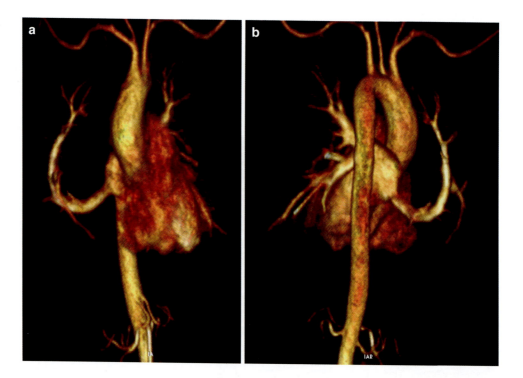

Fig. 51.6. Volume rendered 3D reconstruction of a CE-MRA showing a repaired Scimitar syndrome with redirection of the entire right sided pulmonary venous drainage to the left atrium. (**a**) Anterior and (**b**) posterior views

Notes

52 Ebstein's Anomaly

Describe apical displacement or failure of de-lamination of septal leaflet of tricuspid valve.

Assess mobility of antero-superior & inferior tricuspid valve leaflets – determines feasibility of surgical repair.

Observe presence of eccentric leaflet coaptation.

Quantify tricuspid valve regurgitation.

Quantify RA dilatation and size of atrialized RV.

Assess ventricular function, volumes (LV may be underfilled & compressed, RV may be poorly contractile).

Quantify R-L shunt.

Exclude RVOT obstruction.

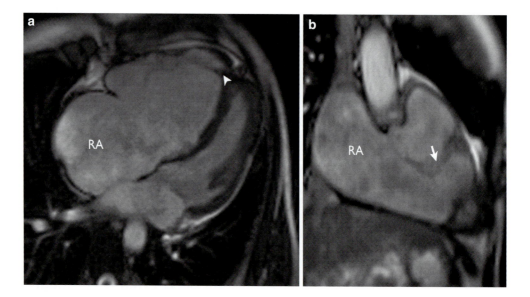

Fig. 52.1. b-SSFP images in a patient with severe Ebstein's anomaly. (**a**) 4-Ch and (**b**) VLA. There is marked apical displacement of the septal leaflet (*arrowhead*), and tethering of the antero-superior leaflet to the right ventricular outflow tract (*arrow*)

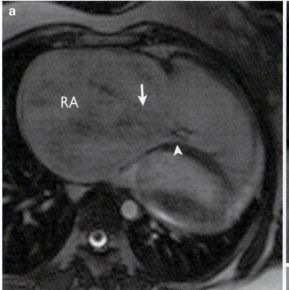

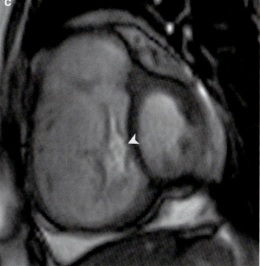

Fig. 52.2. b-SSFP images in a patient with Ebstein's anomaly. (**a**) Oblique axial, (**b**) VLA and (**c**) SA views. There is only mild apical displacement of the septal leaflet, but it is plastered to the interventricular septum with resultant severe tricuspid regurgitation, and a severely dilated right atrium. (**d**) Through-plane phase-contrast velocity image at the level of the tricuspid valve showing severe tricuspid regurgitation

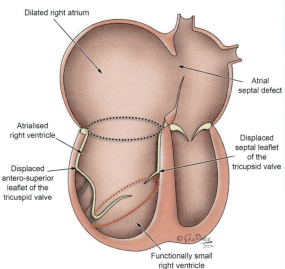

Fig. 52.3. Schematic drawing of Ebstein's Anomaly (4-Ch view)

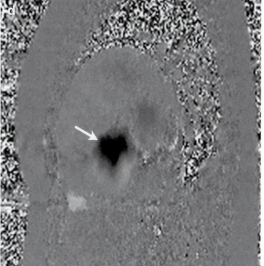

Uhls anomaly – not to be confused

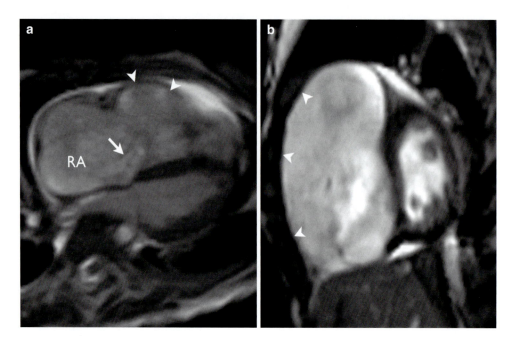

Fig. 52.4. b-SSFP images in a patient with Uhl's anomaly. (**a**) 4-Ch and (**b**) short axis views. The right atrium and ventricle are severely dilated, with thinning of the right ventricular wall (*arrowheads*), and tricuspid regurgitation (*arrow*)

Notes

53 Right Isomerism

Define abdominal, atrial and bronchial situs (Atrial situs alone defines the cardiac isomerism – bilateral R atrial appendages).

Characterise systemic venous (including hepatic) drainage.

Characterise pulmonary venous drainage. Look for TAPVD.

Quantify intracardiac shunt.

Identify any AV valve regurgitation.

Assess ventricular function and volumes.

Look for associated anomalies – large ASD, complete AVSD, DORV, TGA, pulmonary stenosis or atresia.

Consider: intestinal malrotation, large central liver, asplenia, right-sided stomach, bilateral right bronchi and tri-lobar lungs.

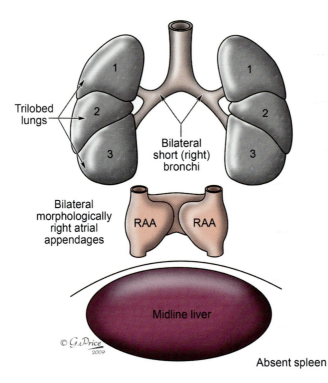

Trilobed lungs

Bilateral short (right) bronchi

Bilateral morphologically right atrial appendages

RAA RAA

Midline liver

© G. Price 2009

Absent spleen

Fig. 53.1. Schematic drawing of right isomerism

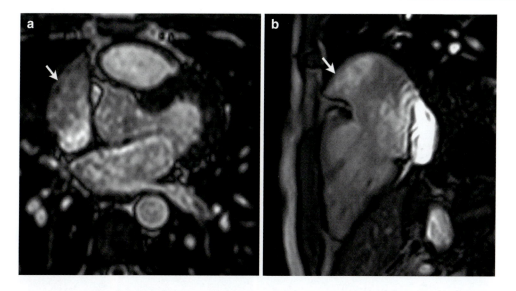

Fig. 53.2. b-SSFP images showing the normal appearance of the right atrial appendage (*arrow*). (**a**) Axial and (**b**) vertical long-axis views

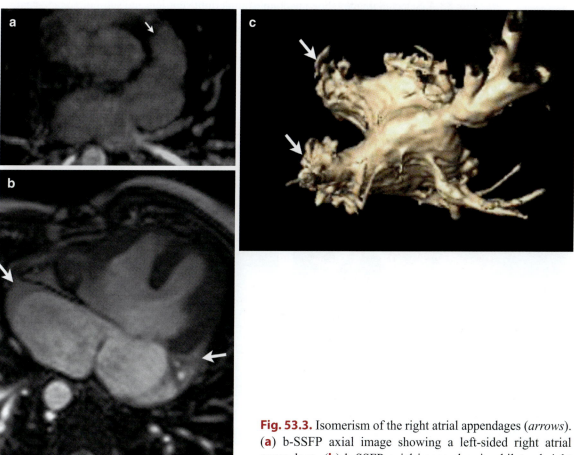

Fig. 53.3. Isomerism of the right atrial appendages (*arrows*). (**a**) b-SSFP axial image showing a left-sided right atrial appendage, (**b**) b-SSFP axial image showing bilateral right atrial appendages and (**c**) volume rendered CE-MRA

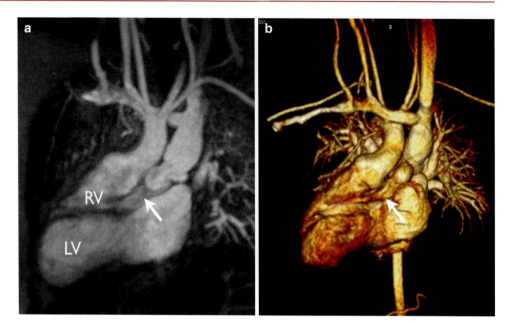

Fig. 53.4. Selected images showing double outlet right ventricle and sub-pulmonary stenosis (*arrow*) in a patient with isomerism of the right atrial appendages. (**a**) 3D b-SSFP and (**b**) volume rendered CE-MRA

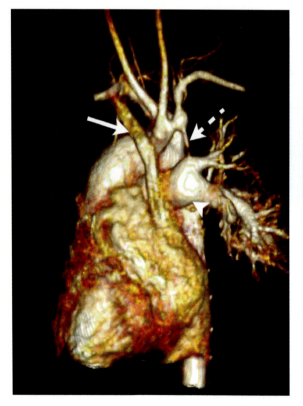

Fig. 53.5. Volume rendered CE-MR angiogram showing a left-sided SVC (*arrow*) draining into a common atrium with absence of the coronary sinus. Also note the post stenotic dilatation of the LPA (*arrowhead*), with a prominent ductus arteriosus (*dashed arrow*)

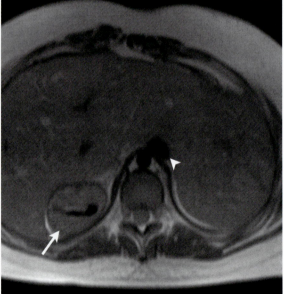

Fig. 53.6. Black blood image showing situs inversus (stomach on the *right arrow*), and an absent spleen. Also note the midline aorta, with the IVC anterior and to the left (*arrowhead*)

Notes

54 Left Isomerism

Define abdominal, atrial and bronchial situs. (Atrial situs alone defines the cardiac isomerism – bilateral L atrial appendages).

Characterise systemic venous drainage – interrupted IVC with azygous continuation.

Characterise pulmonary venous drainage.

Quantify intracardiac shunt.

Identify any AV valve regurgitation.

Assess ventricular function and volumes.

Look for associated anomalies – Large ASD, PAPVD, VSD and DORV.

Consider – intestinal malrotation, biliary atresia, large central liver, polysplenia, bilateral left bronchi and bi-lobar lungs.

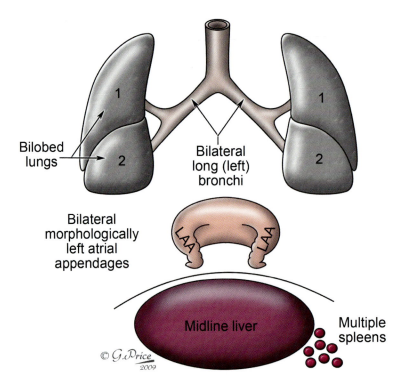

Fig. 54.1. Schematic drawing of left isomerism

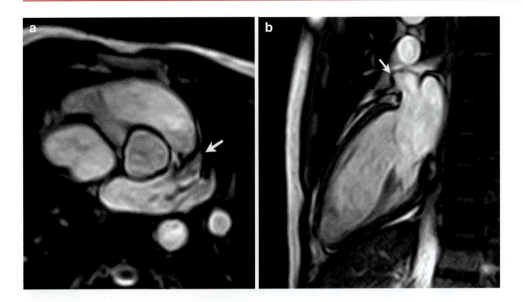

Fig. 54.2. b-SSFP images showing the normal appearance of the left atrial appendage (*arrow*). (**a**) Axial and (**b**) vertical long-axis views

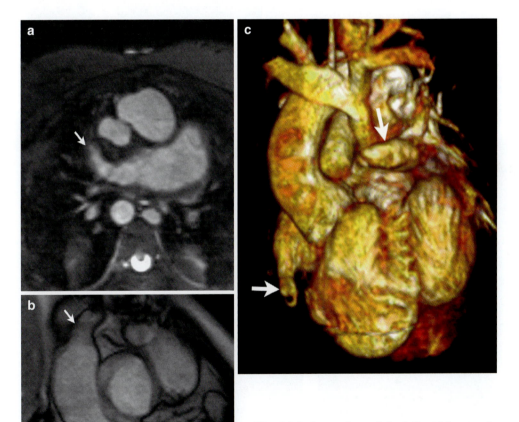

Fig. 54.3. Isomerism of the left atrial appendages (*arrows*). (**a**) Balanced-SSFP axial image showing a right-sided, left atrial appendage. (**b**) Balanced-SSFP axial image showing bilateral left atrial appendages and (**c**) volume rendered CE-MRA showing same (*arrows*)

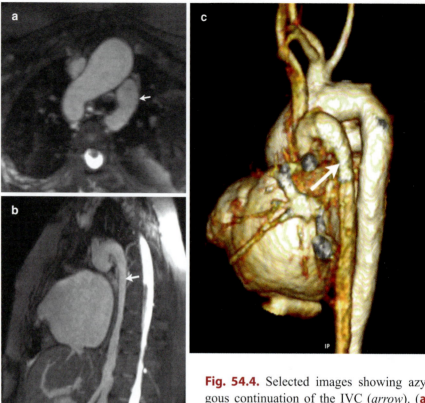

Fig. 54.4. Selected images showing azygous continuation of the IVC (*arrow*). (**a**) Axial MIP image at arch level, (**b**) sagittal MIP image, (**c**) volume rendered CE-MRA

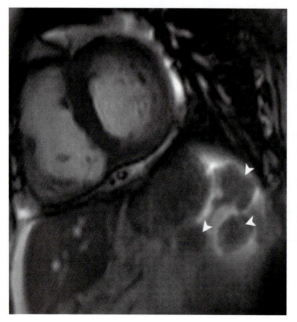

Fig. 54.5. b-SSFP image showing polysplenia (*arrowheads*)

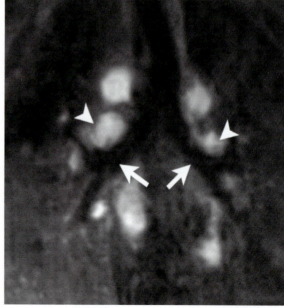

Fig. 54.6. Coronal MinIP from a post CE-MRA showing bilateral left bronchi (*arrows*), and bilateral left pulmonary arteries (*arrowheads*) passing superior to the bronchi

Notes

55 List of Abbreviations

Abbreviations

4-Ch	Four chamber
ALCAPA	Anomalous left coronary artery from the pulmonary artery
AAo	Ascending aorta
Ao	Aorta
AP	Antero-posterior
AR	Aortic regurgitation
ARVC	Arrhythmogenic right ventricular cardiomyopathy
AS	Aortic stenosis
ASD	Atrial septal defect
ASO	Arterial sitch operation
AV	Atrioventricular
AVSD	Atrioventricular septal defect
Azy	Azygous vein
BB	Black blood
BCPC	Bidirectional cavo-pulmonary communication
BCV	Brachiocephalic vein
b-SSFP	Balanced-steady state free precession
BT	Blalock-Taussig
CCTGA	Congenitally corrected transposition of the great arteries
CE	Contrast enhanced
CoA	Coarctation
CT	Computed tomography
CXR	Chest radiograph
DAo	Descending aorta
DILV	Double inlet left ventricle
DKS	Damus-Kaye-Stansel
DORV	Double outlet right ventricle
FF	Forward flow
GA	General anaesthetic
IB	Inferior bridging leaflet (AVSD)
InA	Innominate artery
IR	Inversion recovery
IVC	Inferior vena cava
IVS	Interventricular septum
LA	Left atrium
LAA	Let atrial appendage
LAD	Left anterior descending artery

LCA	Left coronary artery
LCC	Left common carotid artery
LGE	Late gadolinium enhanced
LLPV	Left lower pulmonary vein
LM	Left mural leaflet (AVSD)
LMS	Left main stem
LPA	Left pulmonary artery
LSA	Left subclavian artery
LV	Left ventricle
LVNC	Left ventricular non-compaction
LVOT	Left ventricular outflow tract
LVOTO	Left ventricular outflow tract obstruction
LVSV	Left ventricular stroke volume
MAPCA	Major aortopulmonary collateral arteries
MIP	Maximum intensity projection
MinIP	Minimum intensity projection
MPA	Main pulmonary artery
MPR	Multi planar reformat
MR	Mitral regurgitation
MRI	Magnetic resonance imaging
MRA	Magnetic resonance angiogram
ms	Milliseconds
MV	Mitral valve
PA	Pulmonary artery
PAPVD	Partial anomalous pulmonary venous drainage
PDA	Patent ductus arteriosus
PLE	Protein losing enteropathy
PPVI	Percutaneous pulmonary valve implant
PR	Pulmonary regurgitation notes
PS	Pulmonary stenosis
PT	Pulmonary trunk
Pulm	Pulmonary
PVR	Pulmonary vascular resistance
Qp/Qs	Pulmonary flow/ systemic flow ratio
RA	Right atrium
RAA	Right atrial appendage
RAS	Right anterior superior leaflet (AVSD)
RCA	Right coronary artery
RI	Right inferior leaflet (AVSD)
RLPV	Right lower pulmonary vein

RPA	Right pulmonary artery		TAPVD	Total anomalous pulmonary venous drainage
RV	Right ventricle		TCPC	Total cavo-pulmonary connection
RVOT	Right ventricular outflow tract		TGA	Transposition of the great arteries
RVOTO	Right ventricular outflow tract obstruction		TSE	Turbo spin echo
RVSV	Right ventricular stroke volume		VA	Ventricular-arterial
SA	Short axis		VLA	Vertical long axis
SB	Superior bridging leaflet (AVSD)		VR	Volume rendered
SVC	Superior vena cava		VSD	Ventricular septal defect
SVR	Systemic vascular resistance			

56 Further reading

Anderson RH, Baker EJ, Redington A, Rigby ML (2009) Paediatric Cardiology: Expert Consult. 3rd ed Churchill Livingstone, London

Braunwald E, Gatzoulis MA, Swan L, Therrien J (2005) Adult Congenital Heart Disease: A Practical Guide, 1st ed Wiley-Blackwell, Hoboken, NJ

Bogaert J, Dymarkowski S, Taylor AM (2005) Clinical Cardiac MRI, Springer, Berlin Heidelberg

Lai W, Mertens L, Cohen M, Geva T (2009). Echocardiography In Pediatric and Congenital Heart Disease: From Fetus to Adult, Wiley-Blackwell, Hoboken, NJ

Yagel S, Gembruch U, Silverman NH (2008) Fetal Cardiology: Embryology, Genetics, Physiology, Echocardiography Evaluation, Diagnosis and Perinatal Management of Cardiac Diseases (Series in Maternal Fetal Medicine), 2nd ed Informa Healthcare, London

Printing and Binding: Stürtz GmbH, Würzburg